How to Manage Your Tinnitus

A Step-by-Step Workbook

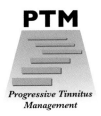

PTM

Progressive Tinnitus Management

How to Manage Your Tinnitus

A Step-by-Step Workbook

James A. Henry
Tara L. Zaugg
Paula J. Myers
Caroline J. Kendall

Illustrations by Lynn F. Kitagawa
Photography by Michael Moody

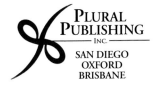

PLURAL
PUBLISHING
INC.

SAN DIEGO
OXFORD
BRISBANE

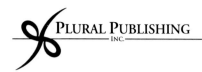

5521 Ruffin Road
San Diego, CA 92123

e-mail: info@pluralpublishing.com
Web site: http://www.pluralpublishing.com

49 Bath Street
Abingdon, Oxfordshire OX14 1EA
United Kingdom

ISBN-13: 978-1-59756-409-0
ISBN-10: 1-59756-409-5

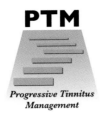

Progressive Tinnitus Management

Acknowledgments

Development and publication of this book was supported by VA Rehabilitation Research and Development (RR&D) Service, the NCRAR, and VA Employee Education System. Numerous individuals have contributed in various and significant ways toward this effort, including:

- **Russell L. Bennett** (Computer Specialist, Long Beach Employee Education Resource Center, Long Beach, California)
- **Daniel C. Garcia** (Graphic Designer, Long Beach Employee Education Resource Center, Long Beach, California)
- **Katie J. Fick, MS** (Research Assistant, James A. Haley Veterans' Hospital, Tampa, Florida)
- **Jeff Hall** (Production Sound Mixer, Salt Lake City Employee Education Resource Center, Salt Lake City, Utah)
- **Christine Kaelin, MBA** (Clinical Research Coordinator, NCRAR, Portland, Oregon)
- **David Lehman** (Executive Producer, Salt Lake City Employee Education Resource Center, Salt Lake City, Utah)
- **Marcia Legro, PhD** (Research Psychologist, Seattle, Washington)
- **Will Murphy** (Audiovisual Production Specialist, Portland VA Medical Center)
- **Kimberly Owens, MPH** (Clinical Research Coordinator, Saint Thomas Research Institute, Nashville, Tennessee)
- **Emily Thielman, MS** (Research Assistant, NCRAR, Portland, Oregon)
- **Dwayne Washington** (Audiovisual Production Specialist, Portland VA Medical Center)
- **John C. Whatley, PhD** (Project Manager, Birmingham Employee Education Resource Center, Birmingham, Alabama)

Also, thanks to Stephen Fausti, PhD and Sara Ruth Oliver, AuD for their continued support of tinnitus research and clinical activities at the Portland VA Medical Center.

Dedication

This book is dedicated to our nation's military veterans. We thank you for serving our country. You are the reason we enjoy freedom.

My Contact Information

Table of Contents

Read Me First

- *This workbook does not, and cannot, provide individual medical advice. It is for general information purposes only. The information is not intended to be a substitute for individual medical advice, diagnosis, or treatment by a physician who is aware of your medical history and has examined you. Do not rely on this workbook in place of seeking professional medical advice.*

- *If you notice any significant change in hearing, tinnitus, or ear-related medical problems, you should contact your primary care provider for referral to an audiologist or ENT (Ear, Nose, Throat) physician, as appropriate. Audiologists do not prescribe medication (drugs). Any medication concerns should be directed to your primary care provider or other physician.*

- *Please contact an audiologist if you have any questions regarding the information contained in this workbook, or if you have questions about tinnitus, hearing loss, or hearing aids.*

- *If you are a Veteran seeking a claim for service connected hearing loss or tinnitus, you should contact your VA Regional Office or Veteran Service Representative for information as to how to proceed.*

- *This workbook presents many different possible ways to manage reactions to tinnitus. In general, VA endorses the method of Progressive Tinnitus Management (PTM). PTM provides a hierarchical structure for providing clinical services for tinnitus. That is, patients should receive services that "progress" to higher levels as needed. Proper evaluation and provision of appropriate education are essential with PTM. Also, PTM is patient-centered and interdisciplinary, consistent with VA's model of health care. However, VA does not endorse any specific device for tinnitus management. Any reference in this workbook (including photographs) to a device does not constitute an endorsement. All of these references are for information purposes only. Also, the methods and devices for managing reactions to tinnitus that are described in this workbook may or may not be available at your regional VA medical center. It is intended that PTM will be available at all VA medical centers in the near future.*

Part 1. Introduction

What is Tinnitus?

Tinnitus is a ringing, humming, buzzing, or other sound in your head or ears that does not have an outside source. The sound comes from within your head. For most people, tinnitus is a constant sound. Tinnitus is not a disease - it is a *symptom*. (See Appendix A for a more complete description of tinnitus.)

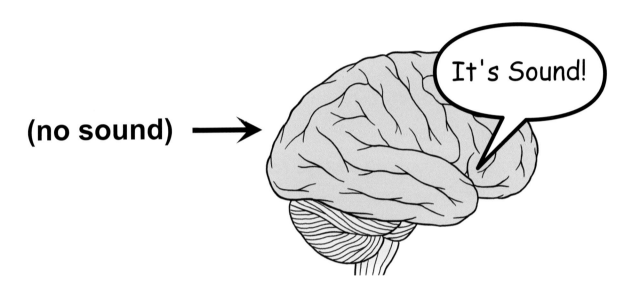

Should I See a Physician?

In most cases, having tinnitus does not mean that you need to see a physician. However, in some cases it is very important to see a physician. If you have tinnitus, you can use the guide below. It will help you decide if you need to see a physician or other health professional.

1 If you experience *any* of the following:

- Injury to your body
- Weakness or paralysis of any muscles in your face
- Sudden unexplained hearing loss in one or both ears

Go to Emergency Care or to an ENT (Ear, Nose, Throat) clinic *immediately*.

2 If you experience *any* of the following:

- Extreme anxiety or depression
- A current plan to end your life and a way to do it

Go to Emergency Care or to a Mental Health clinic *immediately*.

3 If you experience *any* of the following:

- The tinnitus pulses with your heartbeat
- You have ear pain, drainage from your ear, or if there is a foul odor coming from your ear
- You have vertigo (the feeling that you are moving or the room is moving when neither is moving)

Go to an ENT (Ear, Nose, Throat) clinic or to a physician *as soon as possible*.

4 **If you have tinnitus, and** *all* **of the following are true:**

- The tinnitus is a constant sound that does NOT pulse with your heartbeat
- You do NOT have ear pain, drainage from your ear, or foul odor coming from your ear
- You do NOT have vertigo
- You do NOT have weakness or paralysis of any muscles in your face
- You do NOT have sudden unexplained hearing loss

See an audiologist *sometime in the near future.* (An audiologist is a non-physician hearing healthcare provider.)

Tinnitus at a Glance

What Causes Tinnitus?

Anything that causes hearing loss also can cause tinnitus. The most common cause of tinnitus is loud noise. Other causes include:

- Injury to the head or neck
- Various diseases
- Too much ear wax
- Stress
- Prescription drugs

In many cases, there is no known cause. To learn more about causes of tinnitus, see Appendix B.

Can Tinnitus be Cured?

A cure for tinnitus would mean that some treatment could silence it. Although research is being done to find a cure, there is no cure yet. There also is no safe and consistent way to reduce the loudness of tinnitus. We cannot change the tinnitus, but we can change our *reactions* to it. Changing reactions to tinnitus can make it less of a problem. The key is to learn how to *manage* our reactions to tinnitus. The goal is to feel better even though the tinnitus does not change.

Note: In this book we refer to "managing tinnitus." We also refer to "tinnitus management." Both of these terms refer to managing *reactions* to tinnitus. Again, we can't change the loudness of tinnitus, but we can change how we react to it.

How are Reactions to Tinnitus Managed?

Methods that are used in clinics include:

- Sound-based methods (Tinnitus Masking[1], Tinnitus Retraining Therapy[2], Neuromonics Tinnitus Treatment[3])
- Education[4]
- Counseling/Psychotherapy (example: Cognitive-Behavioral Therapy)[5, 6]

Each of these methods has been shown by research to help some people with tinnitus. To learn more about these and other methods, see Appendix C.

Progressive Tinnitus Management

The suggestions in this book are based on the method of Progressive Tinnitus Management (PTM).[7-9] PTM was developed at the National Center for Rehabilitative Auditory Research. The method is "progressive" because not everyone needs the same amount of help. Some people with tinnitus only need basic questions answered. Other people need more than that. Still others need a great deal of help. With PTM, sound is used to manage reactions to tinnitus. However, PTM differs from the sound-based methods listed above. PTM teaches many different ways to use sound to manage tinnitus. Also, PTM teaches ways to change your thoughts and feelings to cope with tinnitus.

What About "Alternative" Methods?

There are many "alternative" methods, including:

- Acupuncture

- Hypnosis

- Vitamins and herbs

- Homeopathy

None of these methods has been shown by research to help people with tinnitus more than placebo.[10] (A placebo is like a "sugar pill.") To learn more about alternative methods, see Appendix C.

Isn't There a Drug for Tinnitus?

All drugs used for tinnitus are meant for other problems - like depression, anxiety, and trouble sleeping.[10] Some of these drugs can improve mood. A better mood can help to make tinnitus less of a problem. In some cases, a drug can reduce the loudness of tinnitus. However, drugs also can make tinnitus *louder*. Any use of drugs for tinnitus involves trial-and-error. Because of possible side effects, the use of drugs should be approached with caution. To learn more about drugs and tinnitus, see Appendix C.

How Can This Workbook Help Me?

There are three basic ways to manage reactions to tinnitus: (1) education and counseling; (2) using sound; and (3) changing thoughts and feelings. These are things that you can do on your own *if you know what to do*. You can learn what to do by reading this workbook.

1. Education

You may have been told in the past to "learn to live with it" and "nothing can be done." This is not true. Doing the activities in this workbook can help you learn to manage your reactions to tinnitus and make it less of a problem.

2. Use of Sound

Most methods of tinnitus management involve *using sound in some way*. Part 2 of this workbook shows you how to use sound to manage reactions to tinnitus.

3. Changing Thoughts and Feelings

In Part 3 of this workbook you will learn:

- Two different ways to relax

- About planning pleasant activities

- How to change your thoughts about tinnitus

All of these are different ways for you to change your thoughts and feelings. Changing your thoughts and feelings can help you manage your reactions to tinnitus.

Goals of Tinnitus Management (All Methods)

There are many methods for managing reactions to tinnitus. These methods are not intended to make your tinnitus quieter. They are intended to help you feel better - even if it's just for a short time - without changing your tinnitus. The more you practice feeling better, the easier it will become to feel OK with your tinnitus just as it is. All of these methods have basically the same goals. They are to:

☐ Feel less stressed about tinnitus

☐ Have fewer emotional reactions to tinnitus

☐ Almost never think about tinnitus

☐ Feel like tinnitus has little effect on daily activities (concentration, work, sleep, etc.)

☐ Feel like tinnitus is not much of a problem

☐ Feel like there is no need for further help learning to manage tinnitus

All of these goals can be accomplished without changing your tinnitus. Go ahead and check the boxes above for the goals that apply to you. Use the space below to write down any other goals you have. Keep in mind that this workbook can help you with tinnitus problems, but not with trouble hearing. For help with trouble hearing, please talk to an audiologist.

_____

_____

_____

_____

_____

_____

What is *your* number one goal for managing your reactions to tinnitus?

_____

_____

_____

_____

Part 2. Step-by-Step Guide: Using Sound to Manage Reactions to Tinnitus

Tinnitus & Hearing Survey

Later on in this workbook, we will be discussing "Bob's" problems with tinnitus and how he learned how to manage them. Bob first filled out the Tinnitus and Hearing Survey. His completed Survey is shown below. Please take a look at how Bob filled out the Survey. Then, answer these questions for yourself on the next page.

Tinnitus and Hearing Survey

Bob

	No, **not** a problem	Yes, a **small** problem	Yes, a **moderate** problem	Yes, a **big** problem	Yes, a **very big** problem	
A. Tinnitus						
Over the last week, tinnitus kept me from sleeping.	0	1	2	③	4	
Over the last week, tinnitus kept me from concentrating on reading.	0	1	②	3	4	
Over the last week, tinnitus kept me from relaxing.	0	①	2	3	4	
Over the last week, I couldn't get my mind off of my tinnitus.	0	1	②	3	4	**Grand Total**
		1	4	3		**8**
Total of each column						
B. Hearing						
Over the last week, I couldn't understand what others were saying in noisy or crowded places.	0	①	2	3	4	
Over the last week, I couldn't understand what people were saying on TV or in movies.	⓪	1	2	3	4	
Over the last week, I couldn't understand people with soft voices.	0	①	2	3	4	
Over the last week, I couldn't understand what was being said in group conversations.	⓪	1	2	3	4	**Grand Total**
		2				**2**
Total of each column						
C. Sound Tolerance						
Over the last week, everyday sounds were too loud for me.*	0	①	2	3	4	
If you responded 1, 2, 3 or 4 to the statement above:						
Being in a meeting with 5 to 10 people would be too loud for me.*	⓪	1	2	3	4	

*If sounds are too loud for you when wearing hearing aids, please tell your audiologist

9

Tinnitus and Hearing Survey

	No, **not** a problem	Yes, a **small** problem	Yes, a **moderate** problem	Yes, a **big** problem	Yes, a **very big** problem
A. Tinnitus					
Over the last week, tinnitus kept me from sleeping.	0	1	2	3	4
Over the last week, tinnitus kept me from concentrating on reading.	0	1	2	3	4
Over the last week, tinnitus kept me from relaxing.	0	1	2	3	4
Over the last week, I couldn't get my mind off of my tinnitus.	0	1	2	3	4

Total of each column

Grand Total

B. Hearing					
Over the last week, I couldn't understand what others were saying in noisy or crowded places.	0	1	2	3	4
Over the last week, I couldn't understand what people were saying on TV or in movies.	0	1	2	3	4
Over the last week, I couldn't understand people with soft voices.	0	1	2	3	4
Over the last week, I couldn't understand what was being said in group conversations.	0	1	2	3	4

Total of each column

Grand Total

C. Sound Tolerance					
Over the last week, everyday sounds were too loud for me.*	0	1	2	3	4

If you responded 1, 2, 3 or 4 to the statement above:

Being in a meeting with 5 to 10 people would be too loud for me.*	0	1	2	3	4

*If sounds are too loud for you when wearing hearing aids, please tell your audiologist

I Completed the Tinnitus and Hearing Survey - What Does it Tell Me?

Sections A and B. Tinnitus problems are managed in a different way than hearing problems. The problems in Section A of the Survey are tinnitus problems. You can use this workbook to learn how to manage tinnitus problems. The problems in Section B are hearing problems. This workbook does not explain how to handle hearing problems. Any hearing professional can help you learn how to manage hearing problems.

Section C. The two questions in section C are about trouble tolerating sound. If you circled any number greater than "0," then read Appendix D. If you circled "2" or greater on the second question, please talk to a hearing professional.

Grand Totals for A and B

- If the Grand Total for A is greater than for B, then you probably *have more trouble with tinnitus than with hearing*.

- If the Grand Total for B is greater than for A, then you probably *have more trouble with hearing than with tinnitus*.

Note: Hearing problems are often helped by hearing aids. Hearing aids can also make tinnitus less of a problem. To learn why hearing aids can be helpful for tinnitus, please see Appendix C.

More Information. See Appendix E to learn more about the effects of tinnitus and why it can be a problem. See Appendix F to learn more about the effects of hearing loss.

Using Sound to Manage Reactions to Tinnitus

In general, there are three *types* of sound that can be used to manage reactions to tinnitus:

1 **Soothing Sound** - *makes you feel better* as soon as you hear it. It helps reduce stress or tension caused by tinnitus.

2 **Background Sound** - *reduces contrast* between tinnitus and a quiet environment. It makes it easier to ignore tinnitus.

3 **Interesting Sound** - *keeps your attention.* It helps shift attention away from tinnitus.

Some types of sound can be used in more than one way at the same time. For example, interesting sound can help to shift attention away from tinnitus. At the same time it can help to reduce stress and tension from tinnitus. Some types of sound can be used in all three ways at the same time. The circles in the figure overlap as a reminder that *the types of sound can overlap.* Regardless of how you use sound, the goal is to help you live with your tinnitus more comfortably. We will now explain each of these three types of sound for managing tinnitus.

Three Types of Sound for Tinnitus

Soothing sound

Soft breezes
Soothing voice
Babbling brook
TINNITUS
Relaxing music
Running water
Ocean waves

ound Other
ther Sound Other
ther Sound Other Sound
ther Sound Other Sound
Other Sound Other Soun
Other Sound Other Soun
Other Sound Other Soun
ther Sound Other Sou
ther Sound Other
ound Other
TINNITUS

Audio Books!
Talk Radio!
TINNITUS
Interesting Music!
Dynamic Speech!

Background sound   **Interesting sound**

Environmental Sound, Music, and Speech

For each type of sound (soothing, background, interesting) you can use environmental sound, music, or speech. Please see the Sound Grid below.

Note: Environmental sound is any sound that is not music or speech. Environmental sounds can be nature sounds (like the sound of ocean waves or insects), or manmade sounds (like fan noise and masking noise).

Sound Grid

The Sound Grid is shown below. It shows that each *type* of sound (soothing, background, interesting) can be environmental sound, music, or speech. This results in nine possible combinations. There is one checkmark on the Sound Grid for each combination.

Sound Grid

	Environmental	Music	Speech
Soothing	✓	✓	✓
Background	✓	✓	✓
Interesting	✓	✓	✓

Soothing Sound

What is Soothing Sound?

- Any sound that makes you feel better as soon as you hear it
- You can use environmental sound, music, or speech as soothing sound

How can Soothing Sound Help?

- By giving you a sense of relief from tension and stress caused by tinnitus

When can I use Soothing Sound?

- Any time your tinnitus bothers you

Soft breezes
Soothing voice
Babbling brook
TINNITUS
Relaxing music
Running water
Ocean waves

Soothing sound

Ernest uses nature sounds from his tabletop sound generator to help him get to sleep. The nature sounds give him a sense of relief from stress and tension caused by tinnitus. The sense of relief makes it easier for him to get to sleep.

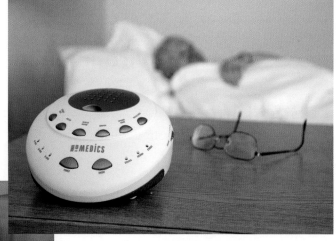

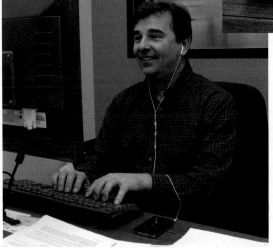

Lee plays recordings of Hawaiian music through his iPod while he is at work. The music gives him a sense of relief from stress and tension caused by his tinnitus. The sense of relief makes it easier for him to concentrate on his work.

Photo of HoMedics sound machine shown with permission from HoMedics, Inc.
Photo of iPod shown with permission from Apple, Inc.

Examples of Soothing Sound

Environmental Sound as Soothing Sound

- Ocean waves
- Wind chimes
- Insect sounds
- Masking noise
- Custom tinnitus-relief sounds
- *Any* environmental sound that is soothing to you

	Environmental	Music	Speech
Soothing	✓		
Background			
Interesting			

Music as Soothing Sound

- Classical music
- New Age music
- Relaxation music
- Music with a slow tempo
- Hawaiian music
- *Any* music that is soothing to you

	Environmental	Music	Speech
Soothing		✓	
Background			
Interesting			

Speech as Soothing Sound

- Recordings of relaxation exercises (Imagery, Deep Breathing, etc.)* (see page 89 in Appendix G)
- Recordings of meditation exercises
- *Any* speech that is soothing to you

	Environmental	Music	Speech
Soothing			✓
Background			
Interesting			

See pages 88-89 in Appendix G for examples of people using soothing sound to manage tinnitus.

*The DVD and the CD in the back of this workbook both have recordings of relaxation exercises (Imagery and Deep Breathing).

Using the Relief Scale for Soothing Sound

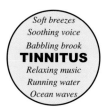

The Relief Scale is shown below. It is used to rate how much relief from stress or tension you feel when you listen to a sound. *No relief* means that there is no change in the stress or tension caused by your tinnitus. *Complete relief* means that, with the sound, the stress or tension caused by the tinnitus is completely gone. Soothing sounds provide a sense of relief from stress or tension caused by tinnitus. You can use the Relief Scale to help you learn which sounds are the most soothing to you. It might take time and patience to find the soothing sounds that do the best job of helping you to feel better.

Instructions:

1 Choose a sound that you think will be soothing. A soothing sound will give you a sense of relief from stress or tension caused by tinnitus. (Tracks 9-14 on the CD in the back of this workbook have sounds that are soothing to many people.)

2 Adjust the volume of the sound until you find the level that is most soothing to you.

3 Answer the question "When I listen to this sound, how much relief from stress and tension do I feel?"

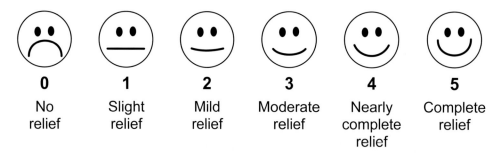

0	1	2	3	4	5
No relief	Slight relief	Mild relief	Moderate relief	Nearly complete relief	Complete relief

Write down the sound that you listened to	How much relief did the sound give you?					
	0	1	2	3	4	5
	0	1	2	3	4	5
	0	1	2	3	4	5
	0	1	2	3	4	5
	0	1	2	3	4	5
	0	1	2	3	4	5

Background Sound

What is Background Sound?

- Any sound that is neutral (not soothing and not interesting)
- You can use environmental sound, music, or speech as background sound

How Can Background Sound Help?

- Our brains are "wired" to notice contrast. There is a lot of contrast between tinnitus and a quiet room. Adding background sound to a quiet room reduces the contrast. The reduced contrast makes it easier to ignore tinnitus.
- Go to pages 19-20 to learn more about *why* background sound makes it easier to ignore tinnitus.

Background sound

When can I use Background Sound?

- Any time your tinnitus bothers you

A constant background of sound can help you notice your tinnitus less often. Background sound should always be set at a comfortable level. The sound should become a natural part of your day. See Appendices G and H for examples of ways to keep a constant background of sound.

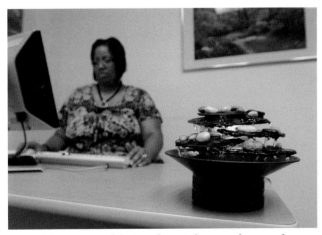

Janet keeps a tabletop fountain running on her desk. The background sound from the fountain makes it easier for her to ignore her tinnitus.

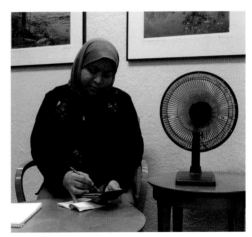

Aynun is using fan noise as background sound to help her concentrate on paying bills.

Photo of tabletop fountain shown with permission from HoMedics, Inc.

Examples of Background Sound

Environmental Sound as Background Sound

- Fan noise
- Waterfall or fountain noise
- Traffic noise
- Wind noise
- Radio static
- Fish tank noise
- *Any* sound that is neutral or pleasant

	Environmental	Music	Speech
Soothing			
Background	✓		
Interesting			

Music as Background Sound

- Classical music
- Guitar or piano music
- New Age music
- Music with lyrics in a foreign language
- "Elevator" music
- *Any* music that is neutral or pleasant

	Environmental	Music	Speech
Soothing			
Background		✓	
Interesting			

Speech as Background Sound

- Recorded crowd noise
- Background television or radio
- *Any* speech that is not interesting to you

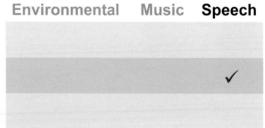

	Environmental	Music	Speech
Soothing			
Background			✓
Interesting			

See pages 90-91 in Appendix G for examples of people using background sound to manage their reactions to tinnitus.

How does Contrast Reduction Make it Easier to Ignore Tinnitus?

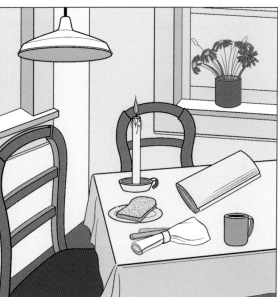

Imagine a lit candle in a dark room. The candle is the only light in the room. There is sharp contrast between the bright candle and the dark room. The candle naturally attracts a lot of attention. Next, imagine the same lit candle, but now with the lights on in the room. The contrast between the candle and the room has been reduced. The candle is just as bright as before, but attracts less attention because now there is other light in the room along with the candle.

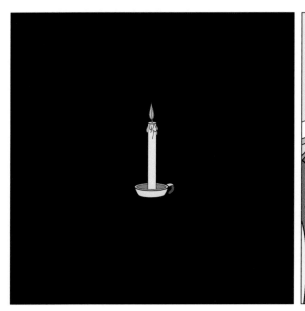

Tinnitus and Background Sound

Contrast reduction also works with sound. The sharp contrast between tinnitus and a quiet room *attracts attention*. Adding sound to the room *reduces the contrast* between the tinnitus and the background. The tinnitus might be just as loud as it was before adding sound to the room. However, *it is easier for the brain to ignore the tinnitus because there is other sound in the room.*

The figure shows how this works. On the left side of the figure "tinnitus" is the only word. When tinnitus is the only word it attracts a lot of attention. On the right side of the figure, there are many words. When there are many words "tinnitus" is easier to ignore, *even though it has not changed.*

Note: Sometimes background sound helps right away. Sometimes it takes weeks or months before you notice that it is helping.

TINNITUS	**ELEVATOR MUSIC** **RADIO STATIC** **CLASSICAL MUSIC** **ELECTRIC FAN** **WHITE NOISE** **GUITAR MUSIC** **TINNITUS** **TRAFFIC NOISE** **WIND NOISE** **AIR CONDITIONER** **NEW AGE MUSIC** **FOUNTAIN NOISE** **FISH TANK NOISE**

Tinnitus Contrast Activity

Instructions:

1. Spend a few moments listening to your tinnitus in quiet.

2. Now turn on some background sound. The sound should be pleasant or neutral. (Tracks 20-23 on the CD in the back of this workbook have sounds that are neutral to many people.)

3. Adjust the volume to a comfortable level.

4. Notice the reduced contrast.

5. Reducing contrast makes it easier to ignore your tinnitus.

TINNITUS	**ELEVATOR MUSIC** **RADIO STATIC** **CLASSICAL MUSIC** **ELECTRIC FAN** **WHITE NOISE GUITAR MUSIC** **TINNITUS** **TRAFFIC NOISE WIND NOISE** **AIR CONDITIONER** **NEW AGE MUSIC** **FOUNTAIN NOISE** **FISH TANK NOISE**

Write down the sound that you listened to	Write any comments you have about using this sound as background sound

Interesting Sound

What is Interesting Sound?

- Sound that keeps your attention
- Sound that you actively listen to
- You can use environmental sound, music, or speech as interesting sound

How can Interesting Sound Help?

- By helping you shift your attention away from your tinnitus

When can Interesting Sound Help?

- When you do not need to concentrate on something else
- When you want to relax or sleep*

*Note: Interesting sound can be a powerful way to get your mind off of your tinnitus. This helps some people relax enough to get to sleep. It might not be helpful for others. Be open to using sound in surprising or unusual ways to manage your tinnitus!

Audio Books!

Talk Radio!

TINNITUS

Interesting Music!

Dynamic Speech!

Interesting sound

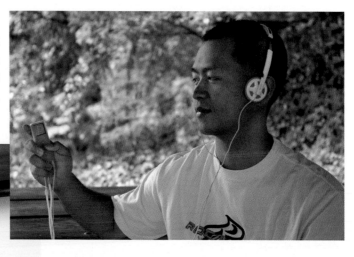

James is listening to an audiobook on his MP3 player. Listening to an audiobook helps him shift his attention away from his tinnitus.

Patrick is talking on the telephone with a friend. Talking on the telephone helps him keep his mind off of his tinnitus.

Examples of Interesting Sound

Environmental Sound as Interesting Sound
Active listening to:

- Whale sounds
- Bird calls
- Morse code
- Forest sounds at night
- *Any* environmental sound that is interesting to you

	Environmental	Music	Speech
Soothing			
Background			
Interesting	✓		

Music as Interesting Sound
Active listening to:

- Song lyrics
- Various instruments in a piece of music
- Live musical performance
- *Any* music that is interesting to you

	Environmental	**Music**	Speech
Soothing			
Background			
Interesting		✓	

Speech as Interesting Sound
Active listening to:

- A friend
- Community lecture
- Audiobook
- Talk radio
- Podcast
- *Any* speech that is interesting to you

	Environmental	Music	**Speech**
Soothing			
Background			
Interesting			✓

See pages 91-92 in Appendix G for examples of people using interesting sound to manage their reactions to tinnitus.

Using the Attention Scale for Interesting Sound

The Attention Scale is shown below. It is used to rate how well a sound keeps your attention off of your tinnitus. You can use the Attention Scale to figure out which sounds work best for keeping your attention. It may take time and patience to find sounds that do the best job of shifting your thoughts away from your tinnitus.

Instructions:

1 Choose a sound that you think will keep your attention. (Tracks 15-19 on the CD in the back of this workbook have sounds that are interesting to many people.)

2 Listen to the sound for at least 1 minute.

3 Choose the percent of attention focused on the sound while listening to it.

Attention focused on:

Tinnitus   Other Sound

0% of attention focused on Other Sound

25% of attention focused on Other Sound

50% of attention focused on Other Sound

75% of attention focused on Other Sound

100% of attention focused on Other Sound

Write down the sound that you listened to	How much of your attention was focused on the "Other Sound"?				
	0%	25%	50%	75%	100%
	0%	25%	50%	75%	100%
	0%	25%	50%	75%	100%
	0%	25%	50%	75%	100%
	0%	25%	50%	75%	100%
	0%	25%	50%	75%	100%

Test Your Understanding

How is Martha Using Sound to Manage Tinnitus?

Challenging Situation: Martha reads a lot of books. She has always enjoyed reading in a quiet area of her house. When her tinnitus started, she felt tense whenever she tried to read there. This made concentration and reading difficult.

Sound Plan: Martha discovered that turning on soft classical music helped her feel less tense and more relaxed. Once she was feeling more relaxed, it was easier for her to concentrate on reading.

Is Martha using . . . Soothing sound? Background sound? Interesting sound?

Answer:
- Soothing sound, because the sound is giving Martha a sense of relief from stress and tension.

- It is also background sound because any use of sound reduces the contrast between the tinnitus and the sound environment.

- It is not interesting sound because she is not paying attention to the sound; also, she should not use interesting sound when reading a book, which requires concentration.

How is Ben Using Sound to Manage Tinnitus?

Challenging Situation: Ben is retired. He likes to relax after breakfast, but is bothered by his tinnitus.

Sound Plan: Ben enjoys listening to bird calls. He can identify many local birds by their calls. After breakfast he sits on his back porch and listens to bird calls. Other times he goes on-line to learn new bird calls. Listening to bird calls is interesting to Ben, and helps to get his mind off of his tinnitus.

Is Ben using . . . Soothing sound? Background sound? Interesting sound?

Answer:
- Interesting sound, because Ben actively listens to the sound, which takes his mind off of his tinnitus.

- It is also background sound because any use of sound reduces the contrast between tinnitus and the sound environment.

- It may also be soothing sound if Ben feels a sense of relief from stress and tension; this is not clear from the information provided.

How is Betty Using Sound to Manage Tinnitus?

Challenging Situation: Betty works at home. She spends most of her day working on the computer. The room is very quiet and her tinnitus makes it hard for her to concentrate. She tried playing music, but it was too distracting.

Sound Plan: She then tried opening the window. She could hear traffic noise from the freeway, which reduced the contrast between her tinnitus and the quiet room without creating a distraction. It is now easier for her to concentrate on her work.

Is Betty using . . . Soothing sound? Background sound? Interesting sound?
Answer:
  • Background sound, because it is neither soothing nor interesting to Betty.

Video: "Managing Your Tinnitus: What To Do and How To Do It"

There is a video on DVD that came with this workbook ("Managing Your Tinnitus: What To Do and How To Do It.") The video has two sessions that teach how sound is used to manage reactions to tinnitus. It also shows how to develop a personal "sound plan," which is described in the next section of this workbook. The video may help you to understand these concepts. Try to watch the video at least once. If you do not have a DVD player, you can use the instructions in this workbook instead - or go to your public library to view the video.

Develop a Personal "Sound Plan"

The Sound Plan Worksheet provides step-by-step instructions to create your own "sound plan" to manage your tinnitus. (An example of a completed Sound Plan Worksheet is shown on page 30.) Use the Tinnitus Problem Checklist (p. 29) to list up to three situations when your tinnitus is bothersome. For each situation that you list, use a separate Sound Plan Worksheet. (Blank Worksheets are provided at the end of this workbook.) Each Worksheet helps you to develop a "plan of action" to use sound to manage your reactions to tinnitus. Try each plan of action for 1 week. Then note on the Worksheet how helpful it was.

Key Points for Your First Sound Plan Worksheet

Your first plan should be something you can do easily on your own. Create a plan using **sounds** and **sound sources** that *you already have*.

- **Sounds** can be any kind of environmental sound, music, or speech
- **Sound sources** can include CD players, tabletop fountains, radios, electric fans - anything that creates a sound (see Appendix H for ideas)

As you try your first plan, you will begin learning what is helpful for you.

- You can then make changes to improve your plan

Ongoing Use of the Sound Plan Worksheet

It takes trial and error to learn what works best in each situation. Use the Worksheet on a regular basis to change and improve your sound plans. Also, use the Worksheet to create new sound plans for different situations. Continue using the Worksheet for as long as your tinnitus is a problem.

How to Fill Out the Sound Plan Worksheet

See the example of a completed Sound Plan Worksheet on page 30. The example Worksheet was completed for "Bob," who is described below.

Bob

Bob had trouble falling asleep at night because he was annoyed by the sound of his tinnitus in his quiet bedroom. He tried listening to books on CD, but that was not helpful. He tried watching television. That was only a little helpful. Then he tried listening to talk radio. That was very helpful.

He now listens to talk radio while falling asleep at night. Listening to the radio helps to keep his mind off of his tinnitus so that he can relax enough to get to sleep. He uses a small portable radio connected to earbuds. The radio turns off automatically after 60 minutes. He usually falls asleep with the earbuds still in his ears. He removes the earbuds when he wakes up.

Listening to talk radio helped Bob get to sleep at night. But when he woke up in the middle of the night, he did not want to listen to the radio. He decided to purchase a box fan that he placed next to his bed. The sound of the fan reduces the contrast between his tinnitus and the quiet environment. This makes it easier to fall back to sleep.

Tinnitus Problem Checklist

1. My **most** bothersome tinnitus situation is:

☐ Falling asleep at night   ☐ Relaxing in my recliner

☐ Staying asleep at night   ☐ Napping during the day

☐ Waking up in the morning   ☐ Planning activities

☐ Reading   ☐ Driving

☐ Working at the computer   ☐ Other _____

Now, write your answer on #1 of the Sound Plan Worksheet. (Copies of the Worksheet can be found at the end of this workbook.)

2. My **second most** bothersome tinnitus situation is:

☐ Falling asleep at night   ☐ Relaxing in my recliner

☐ Staying asleep at night   ☐ Napping during the day

☐ Waking up in the morning   ☐ Planning activities

☐ Reading   ☐ Driving

☐ Working at the computer   ☐ Other _____

Now, write your answer on #1 of a *separate* Sound Plan Worksheet.

3. My **third most** bothersome tinnitus situation is:

☐ Falling asleep at night   ☐ Relaxing in my recliner

☐ Staying asleep at night   ☐ Napping during the day

☐ Waking up in the morning   ☐ Planning activities

☐ Reading   ☐ Driving

☐ Working at the computer   ☐ Other _____

Now, write your answer on #1 of a *separate* Sound Plan Worksheet.

Sound Plan Worksheet

Bob

1. Write down one bothersome tinnitus situation _falling asleep at night_

2. **Check one or more** of the three ways to use sound to manage the situation

3. **Write down the sounds** that you will try

4. **Write down the devices** you will use

5. Use your sound plan **over the next week. How helpful** was each sound after using it for 1 week?

6. **Comments** When you find something that works well (or not so well) please comment. You do not need to wait 1 week to write your comments.

☐ **Soothing sound**

(TINNITUS circle: Soft breezes / Soothing voice / Bubbling brook / Relaxing music / Running water / Ocean waves)

	Not at all	A little	Moderately	Very much	Extremely
	☐	☐	☐	☐	☐

☑ **Background sound**

(TINNITUS circle: Sound Other / Other Sound Other / Other Sound Other Sound / Other Sound Only / Sound Other)

fan — _box fan_

	Not at all	A little	Moderately	Very much	Extremely
	☐	☐	☑	☐	☐

adding fan noise helped me get to sleep and helped me stay asleep

☑ **Interesting sound**

(TINNITUS circle: Talk Radio! / TINNITUS / Audio Books!)

television — _TV in bedroom_
talk radio — _radio with earbuds_
books on CD — _CD player by bed with earbuds_

	Not at all	A little	Moderately	Very much	Extremely
	☐	☑	☐	☑	☐

talk radio helped me get to sleep but I still wake up in the night

30

How do I fill out #1 on the Sound Plan Worksheet?

Sound Plan Worksheet

1. Write down one bothersome tinnitus situation _____

2. **Check one or more** of the three ways to use sound to manage the situation	3. **Write down the sounds** that you will try	4. **Write down the devices** you will use	5. Use your sound plan **over the next week. How helpful** was each sound after using it for 1 week?	6. **Comments** When you find something that works well (or not so well) please comment. You do not need to wait 1 week to write your comments.
☐ **Soothing sound** (Soft breezes, Soothing voice, Babbling brook, TINNITUS, Relaxing music, Running water, Ocean waves)	_____ _____ _____	_____ _____ _____	Not at all / A little / Moderately / Very much / Extremely ☐☐☐☐☐ ☐☐☐☐☐ ☐☐☐☐☐	_____ _____ _____
☐ **Background sound** (Sound Other... TINNITUS... Sound Oth...)	_____ _____ _____	_____ _____ _____	Not at all / A little / Moderately / Very much / Extremely ☐☐☐☐☐ ☐☐☐☐☐ ☐☐☐☐☐	_____ _____ _____
☐ **Interesting sound** (Talk Radio!, TINNITUS, Audio Books!)	_____ _____ _____	_____ _____ _____	Not at all / A little / Moderately / Very much / Extremely ☐☐☐☐☐ ☐☐☐☐☐ ☐☐☐☐☐	_____ _____ _____

First, fill out the Tinnitus Problem Checklist (page 29).

Write one bothersome situation from the Tinnitus Problem Checklist at the top of the Worksheet (#1). (see below)

- If this is your first time filling out the Worksheet, use #1 from the Checklist.
- Fill out a separate Worksheet for each problem listed on the Tinnitus Problem Checklist.

Tinnitus Problem Checklist

1. My **most** bothersome tinnitus situation is:

☑ Falling asleep at night   ☐ Relaxing in my recliner
☐ Staying asleep at night   ☐ Napping during the day
☐ Waking up in the morning   ☐ Planning activities
☐ Reading   ☐ Driving
☐ Working at the computer   ☐ Other _____

Now, write your answer on #1 of the Sound Plan Worksheet. (Copies of the Worksheet can be found at the end of this workbook.)

2. My **second most** bothersome tinnitus situation is:

☐ Falli...
☐ Stay...
☐ Wak...
☑ Rea...
☐ Worl...

Now, wr...

3. My th...

☐ Falli...
☐ Stay...
☐ Wak...
☐ Rea...
☐ Worl...

Now, wr...

Sound Plan Worksheet

Bob

1. Write down one bothersome tinnitus situation _falling asleep at night_

2. **Check one or more** of the three ways to use sound to manage the situation	3. **Write down the sounds** that you will try	4. **Write down the devices** you will use	5. Use your sound plan **over the next week.** How helpful was each sound after using it for 1 week?	6. **Comments** When you find something that works well (or not so well) please comment. You do not need to wait 1 week to write your comments.
☐ Soothing sound (Soft breezes / Soothing voice / Bubbling brook / TINNITUS / Relaxing music / Running water / Ocean waves)			Not at all / A little / Moderately / Very much / Extremely	
☑ Background sound (Other Sound Other So... / TINNITUS / Other Sound Other So...)	fan	box fan	☐ ☐ ☑ ☐ ☐ (Moderately)	adding fan noise helped me get to sleep and helped me stay asleep
☑ Interesting sound (Talk Radio! / TINNITUS / Audio Books!)	television / talk radio / books on CD	Tv in bedroom / radio with earbuds / CD player by bed with earbuds	☐ ☑ ☐ ☐ ☐ (A little); ☐ ☐ ☐ ☑ ☐ (Very much); ☑ ☐ ☐ ☐ ☐ (Not at all)	talk radio helped me get to sleep, but I still wake up in the night

How do I fill out #2 on the Sound Plan Worksheet?

For #2 of the Worksheet, check one, two, or all three types of sound. Choose types of sound that you think will help you with the problem listed in #1 of the Worksheet. If the problem you listed requires concentration, then do not choose interesting sound.

- A description of soothing sound is on page 14

- A description of background sound is on page 17

- A description of interesting sound is on page 22

- Sample recordings of soothing, background, and interesting sounds are on the CD in the back of this workbook.

Sound Plan Worksheet

1. Write down one bothersome tinnitus situation _____

2. **Check one or more** of the three ways to use sound to manage the situation	3. **Write down the sounds** that you will try	4. **Write down the devices** you will use	5. Use your sound plan **over the next week. How helpful** was each sound after using it for 1 week?	6. **Comments** When you find something that works well (or not so well) please comment. You do not need to wait 1 week to write your comments.
☐ **Soothing sound** *Soft breezes* *Soothing voice* *Babbling brook* **TINNITUS** *Relaxing music* *Running water* *Ocean waves*	_____ _____ _____	_____ _____ _____	Not at all / A little / Moderately / Very much / Extremely ☐ ☐ ☐ ☐ ☐ ☐ ☐ ☐ ☐ ☐ ☐ ☐ ☐ ☐ ☐	_____ _____ _____
☐ **Background sound** *Sound Other* *ther Sound Other Soun* **TINNITUS** *Other Sound Other Sou* *d Other Sound Oth* *ound Othe*	_____ _____ _____	_____ _____ _____	Not at all / A little / Moderately / Very much / Extremely ☐ ☐ ☐ ☐ ☐ ☐ ☐ ☐ ☐ ☐ ☐ ☐ ☐ ☐ ☐	_____ _____ _____
☐ **Interesting sound** *Talk* *Radio!* **TINNITUS** *Audio* *Books!*	_____ _____ _____	_____ _____ _____	Not at all / A little / Moderately / Very much / Extremely ☐ ☐ ☐ ☐ ☐ ☐ ☐ ☐ ☐ ☐ ☐ ☐ ☐ ☐ ☐	_____ _____ _____

How do I fill out #3 on the Sound Plan Worksheet?

For each type of sound that you chose for #2, write the specific sounds that you will try.

- Ideas for soothing sound are on pages 14-15 and 88-89
- Ideas for background sound are on pages 17-18 and 90-91
- Ideas for interesting sound are on pages 22-23 and 91-92

Bob

Sound Plan Worksheet

1. Write down one bothersome tinnitus situation _falling asleep at night_

2. **Check one or more** of the three ways to use sound to manage the situation	3. **Write down the sounds** that you will try	4. **Write down the devices** you will use	5. Use your sound plan **over the next week**. How helpful was each sound after using it for 1 week?	6. **Comments** When you find something that works well (or not so well) please comment. You do not need to wait 1 week to write your comments.
☐ **Soothing sound** *Soft breezes Soothing voice Babbling brook* **TINNITUS** *Relaxing music Running water Ocean waves*	_____ _____ _____	_____ _____ _____	Not at all / A little / Moderately / Very much / Extremely (EXAMPLE)	_____ _____ _____
☑ **Background sound** *Sound Other So... er Sound Other Sou* **TINNITUS** *Other Sound Other So... d Other Sound Oth... ound Oth...*	_fan_ _____ _____	_box fan_ _____	Moderately ☑	_adding fan noise helped me get to sleep and helped me stay asleep_
☑ **Interesting sound** **Talk Radio!** **TINNITUS** **Audio Books!**	_television_ _talk radio_ _books on CD_	_TV in bedroom_ _radio with earbuds_ _CD player by bed with earbuds_	A little ☑ Very much ☑ Not at all ☑	_talk radio helped me get to sleep, but I still wake up in the night_

How do I fill out #4 on the Sound Plan Worksheet?

For each **sound** that you listed under #3, write in the **device(s)** you will use.

- If this is your first time filling out a Worksheet, write in devices that you already have

- Once you have used the Worksheet at least once, you can start thinking about using devices you do not yet own

- Appendix H gives ideas for devices to use as sources of sound

Bob

Sound Plan Worksheet

1. Write down one bothersome tinnitus situation _falling asleep at night_

2. **Check one or more** of the three ways to use sound to manage the situation	3. **Write down the sounds** that you will try	4. **Write down the devices** you will use	5. Use your sound plan **over the next week. How helpful** was each sound after using it for 1 week?	6. **Comments** When you find something that works well (or not so well) please comment. You do not need to wait 1 week to write your comments.
☐ **Soothing sound**			Not at all / A little / Moderately / Very much / Extremely	
☑ **Background sound**	fan	box fan	☑ Moderately	adding fan noise helped me get to sleep and helped me stay asleep
☑ **Interesting sound**	television / talk radio / books on CD	Tv in bedroom / radio with earbuds / CD player by bed with earbuds	☑ A little / ☑ Very much / ☑ Not at all	talk radio helped me get to sleep, but I still wake up in the night

EXAMPLE

How do I fill out #5 on the Worksheet?

- Use your sound plan for at least one week

- Rate each sound after trying it for at least one week

- Use the ratings under #5 to help guide changes and improvements in your plan

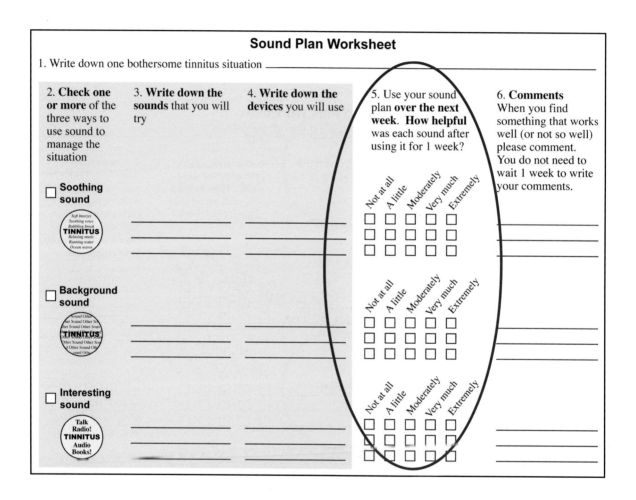

Sound Plan Worksheet

1. Write down one bothersome tinnitus situation _____

2. **Check one or more** of the three ways to use sound to manage the situation	3. **Write down the sounds** that you will try	4. **Write down the devices** you will use	5. Use your sound plan **over the next week**. How helpful was each sound after using it for 1 week?	6. **Comments** When you find something that works well (or not so well) please comment. You do not need to wait 1 week to write your comments.

Part 3. Step-by-Step Guide: Changing Thoughts and Feelings to Manage Reactions to Tinnitus

Many people put a lot of time, effort, and money into trying to quiet their tinnitus. This is normal because quieting the tinnitus would solve the problem. However, there is no cure for tinnitus for most people. Usually the more people try to quiet their tinnitus, the more frustrated they become. In spite of all of their efforts they usually end up feeling worse.

There are many ways to feel better without quieting your tinnitus. You've already learned about three types of sound you can use to manage your reactions to tinnitus. Using sound is something you can *do* to help you feel better. Using sound is a *behavior*.

In this chapter, you will now learn more behaviors to manage your reactions to tinnitus, including:

1 Practicing **relaxation exercises**
2 Increasing **pleasant activities**
3 Learning how to **change your thoughts** about your tinnitus

These may be new behaviors for you. You can learn and practice these new behaviors. Then you will have new skills to manage your reactions to tinnitus.

Note about sleep: Getting enough sleep can help you feel better and think more clearly. Getting enough sleep can make it easier for you to manage your tinnitus. Appendix I gives tips for getting better sleep.

Relaxation Exercises

Many people with tinnitus say stress makes their tinnitus worse. Relaxation exercises can reduce stress. These exercises can slow down your breathing and reduce your heart rate. This workbook provides instructions for two relaxation exercises:

1 Deep Breathing
2 Imagery

---

breathe

Relax

imagine

Relaxation exercises

What is Deep Breathing?

• Focusing on your breathing to help you relax

What is Imagery?

• Imagining a calming and peaceful place

How can Deep Breathing and Imagery Help?

• By slowing down your body

• By helping you get your mind off of your tinnitus[5]

• By helping you feel relaxed and calm

   - Feeling relaxed and calm can help you:

      Feel a sense of relief from tension and stress caused by tinnitus

      Think more clearly and function better

      Feel better overall

When can I use Deep Breathing and Imagery?

• Any time you feel stressed or tense

Prepare to begin Deep Breathing and Imagery

1 Find a relaxing place where you will not be disturbed. If needed, take the phone off the hook and ask others to give you this time alone. Loosen any tight clothing or change into comfortable clothes.

2 Sit in a chair with your feet flat on the floor or propped up. Place your hands in your lap or on the arms of the chair. Make sure you are comfortable.

3 Turn on a soothing sound. Avoid silence while you are practicing deep breathing or imagery. You might have a soothing sound on your Sound Plan (from Part 2 of this workbook) that you can use. If not, turn on music or other sound that helps you feel calm. If you prefer, you can use background sound while you are deep breathing.

Deep Breathing Instructions Step-by-Step

1 Prepare to begin by following steps 1-3 above

2 Place one hand on your stomach and one hand on your chest. Take a normal breath in and notice which hand moves the most. Most likely it will be the hand on your chest. This shows that you tend to breathe shallow breaths from your chest. Now try to take a breath from your abdomen (stomach). You might feel like you are pushing your stomach out - that is how it feels when you are more relaxed and breathing more deeply.

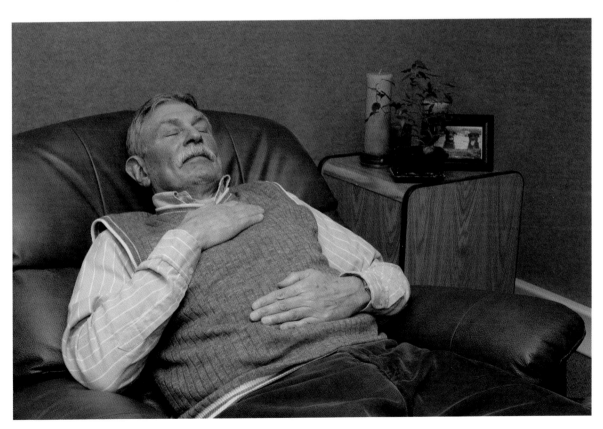

3 Close your eyes (if you are comfortable doing so) or look at an object in the room like a book on the bookshelf

4 Take a deep breath in through your nose - slowly for a count of three. (Remember to use your stomach first and let your chest expand naturally after that.)

5 Hold that breath for two seconds and then exhale for a count of three from your mouth

6 Repeat steps 4 and 5 at least five times

7 When you are ready to stop the Deep Breathing exercise, count back from 3 to 1:

   3 - Become aware of your surroundings

   2 - Move your feet, legs, hands, arms, and rotate your head

   1 - Open your eyes feeling relaxed

Imagery

Choose a Calming and Peaceful Place to Imagine

Before you begin, choose a place you will imagine. You can imagine any place that would be calming and peaceful for you. You should feel safe there.

When you are choosing what you will imagine, think about these things:

- **The place:** Where do you want to be?
  Examples: the beach or in your kitchen

- **Sight:** What do you see?
  Examples: trees, grass, the sun, or an oven

- **Smell:** What do you smell?
  Examples: the ocean, pine, flowers, or cooking food

- **Sounds:** What do you hear?
  Examples: birds, twigs cracking, soft waves, or boiling water

- **Touch:** What do you feel?
  Examples: a cool breeze, the warm sun, or heat from cooking

- **Taste:** What can you taste?
  Examples: salty air, sweet berries, cool water, or warm food

Imagery Instructions Step-by-Step

1   Prepare to begin by following steps 1 through 3 on page 38

2   Take several deep breaths and shift your focus to the peaceful image you chose.

3   As you focus your thoughts on your peaceful place:
   - Imagine a path you travel on as you journey through your place.
     Example: As you look back notice your footprints in the sand where you have just walked along the shore. Slowly, a wave moves in and washes away the sand.
   - Imagine what you hear, smell, and taste.
   - Imagine reaching out and touching things around you.
     Example: Notice how the sand or a leaf feels as you hold it in your hand.
   - As you imagine your relaxing place, move deeper and deeper into the image. You should feel calm and peaceful there.
   - Notice how your body feels - you will want to return to this feeling next time.

4   When you are ready to stop imagining the peaceful place, count back from 3 to 1:

   3 - Become aware of your surroundings

   2 - Move your feet, legs, hands, arms, and rotate your head

   1 - Open your eyes feeling relaxed

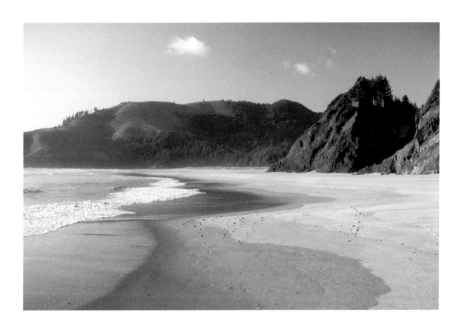

Practice Video: Deep Breathing and Imagery

There is a video on the DVD that came with this workbook ("Managing Your Tinnitus, Deep Breathing Exercise"). It shows a man using deep breathing to relax. Later, he uses imagery to relax when his tinnitus is bothering him at work. You can watch the video to learn deep breathing and imagery. Try to watch the video at least once. You can keep using the video while you practice, or you can begin doing the exercises on your own. If you do not have a DVD player, you can use the instructions in this workbook instead - or go to your public library to view the video.

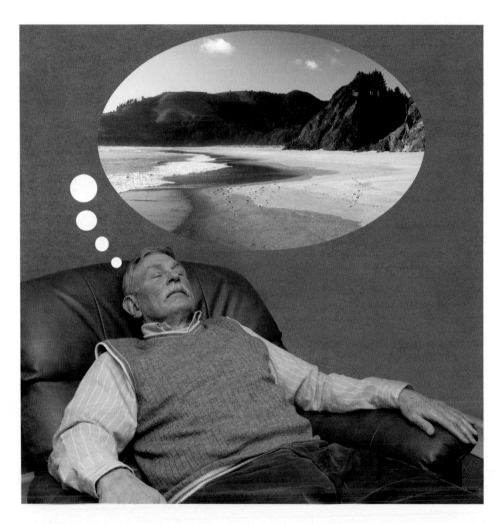

Relief Scale

The Relief Scale is shown below. Use it to rate how much relief from stress or tension you feel after using deep breathing or imagery. *No relief* means that there is no change in the stress or tension caused by your tinnitus. *Complete relief* means that the stress or tension caused by the tinnitus is completely gone. Learning to relax using deep breathing and imagery takes time and practice. You can use the Relief Scale to track your progress.

Instructions

- Get into a comfortable position
- Follow the instructions for deep breathing (p. 39) or imagery (p. 41)
- Fill out the chart below to track your progress

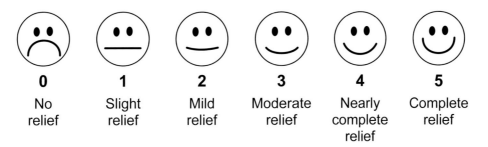

0	1	2	3	4	5
No relief	Slight relief	Mild relief	Moderate relief	Nearly complete relief	Complete relief

| Date | Time of Day | Minutes Practiced | | Relief |
		Deep Breathing	Imagery	
Example: June 5, 2009	10:00am	5 mins	0	3
June 5, 2009	10:05am	0	5 mins	4

Pleasant Activity Scheduling

What are pleasant activities?

• Activities you *enjoy*

• Activities you *like* to do but do not *have* to do

How can pleasant activities help me manage my reactions to tinnitus?

• By helping you have more positive feelings

• By distracting you from your tinnitus

• By helping you feel better overall

golf, write, walk

Pleasant activities

dance, paint

Plan pleasant activities

What You <u>Do</u> Affects How You <u>Feel</u>

Some people with tinnitus feel like they can't enjoy life again unless the tinnitus is quieter or gone. Because of this, they may stop doing many of their usual activities - especially activities they enjoy. If *you* are doing fewer activities because of tinnitus, then you are more likely to be focused on your tinnitus, and you are more likely to feel unhappy. [Note: If you are stopping activities because of trouble hearing, then that is a separate concern - please see Appendix F.]

One way to start feeling better is to plan pleasant activities even when your tinnitus is bothering you. Pleasant activities can help you enjoy life and pay less attention to your tinnitus. At first, you might feel like you are "relearning" how to enjoy pleasant activities. The activities might be harder to enjoy than they were without tinnitus. With time, you can learn to enjoy the activities even with tinnitus.

Activity Planning

What kinds of activities fill your day? Are they all tasks you feel you "have to do?" Do you have any activities you enjoy during the day?

One way to increase pleasant activities is to *plan ahead*. This may sound simple, but most of the time we wait until we feel better to do something we enjoy. If you let *how you feel* guide *what you do*, then you may end up staying home and not doing anything. If you schedule pleasant activities you will find it easier to do something you enjoy. As a result, you may feel more pleasure!

We will ask you to keep track of your activities. This will help you be aware of how you spend each day. Once you see what you are doing now, then you can begin to change or increase your pleasant activities.

Consider these specific categories of activities during the upcoming week:

1   Activities you feel you *have* to do
2   Activities you *like* to do

Increasing Pleasant Activities - Step-by-Step:

Step 1: Track Your Activities. Use the "Track Your Activities" worksheet below. When you do an activity, write it down along with the day and time. Then, choose from the two categories of activities:

1   Activities you *have* to do
2   Activities you *like* to do

This shows the kinds of activities you are doing. If you don't see many #2's then you need more pleasant activities in your life! Plan at *least* one pleasant activity each day.

Step 2: Make a List of Pleasant Activities. Identify pleasant activities that *you* would enjoy. Use the "Make a List of Pleasant Activities" form below. Choose 10 pleasant activities that you would enjoy. These activities can be with other people or by yourself. Make sure that the activity is pleasant for you.

Step 3: Plan Pleasant Activities. Sometimes it's hard to fit everything you want to do into your schedule. Unless you plan the activity by scheduling it, you may continue with your routine as it is. Try to plan at least one pleasant activity per day by using your own calendar or scheduler. Write down how long you will do the activity and when you will do it. These activities can be done alone or with other people. Just be sure the activity is pleasant for you.

Step 1: Track Your Activities. Directions: Write down your activities over the next 6 days. Fill in the **Day** of the week, the **Activity** during each **Time** frame, and the **Category** of the activity.

Day	Time	Activity	Activity Category *Have to do = 1* *Like to do = 2*
Example: **Day 1** *Monday*	Morning	Example: *Went to work*	I
	Afternoon	Example: *Still at work, worked out at the gym*	I, I
	Evening	Example: *Made dinner, cleaned up the kitchen, watched TV*	I, I, 2
Day 1	Morning		
	Afternoon		
	Evening		
Day 2	Morning		
	Afternoon		
	Evening		
Day 3	Morning		
	Afternoon		
	Evening		
Day 4	Morning		
	Afternoon		
	Evening		
Day 5	Morning		
	Afternoon		
	Evening		
Day 6	Morning		
	Afternoon		
	Evening		

Total #1's = _____

Total #2's = _____

Step 2: Make a List of Pleasant Activities. Before you can plan pleasant activities, you first need to know what activities you would enjoy. Below are some types of pleasant activities. List only activities you would enjoy.

Type of Activity	Example Activity	Activity
Social	Dinner with friends	
Recreational	Taking dance lessons	
Sporting	Playing golf	
Creative	Writing poetry	
Educational	Taking a history class	
Solitary	A walk in the woods	
Artistic	Painting	
Pampering	Getting a massage	
Musical	Playing the piano	
Interest-oriented	Collecting old cameras	
Travel	Going to Hawaii	
Food	Baking bread	

[Note: these categories adapted from JL Henry and Wilson[6]]

Step 3: Plan Pleasant Activities. The last step is to plan your activities. On your own calendar write down one pleasant activity you will do each day. After you do this for 1 week, look back at days when you did not do a pleasant activity. Ask yourself:

1   Did I do all of my scheduled pleasant activities each day?

2   Why didn't I do some or all of my activities as planned?

3   Did I notice my tinnitus less when I did these activities?

4   Would more activities help me get my mind off of my tinnitus?

5   Do I need to have more or fewer pleasant activities?

Changing Thoughts

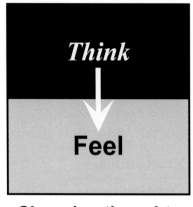

Changing thoughts

What does "Changing Thoughts" mean?

- First you identify thoughts you had just before feeling bad

- Then you work on changing that thought to something that is more helpful

How can "Changing Thoughts" help?

- Changing your thoughts about tinnitus can help you change the way you feel about it

When can I use "Changing Thoughts"?

- Any time you feel tension or stress when you think about your tinnitus

Thoughts Affect Feelings

What you *think* affects how you *feel*. For example, imagine you are expecting guests to come to your house for dinner and they don't show up on time. The thoughts you have about your guests being late will affect how you feel (your emotions). If you think "it's rude to be late," then you might get *angry*. If you think "it's nice to have extra time to clean up," then you may feel *relieved*. If you think "they could have been in an accident," then you might become *worried*. In this example, the event is the same, but your thoughts about the event are different. Sometimes the way you feel is caused by the *thoughts* about the event, not the event itself.

What thoughts do you have about your tinnitus? When you think about tinnitus, how do you feel?

Feelings Affect Health

What you think affects how you feel, and your feelings affect your health. Stress and negative emotions can lead to many health problems.[2] In times of stress our brains release hormones into our bodies. These hormones increase heart rate, blood pressure, and muscle tension. The changes caused by these hormones help us react to emergencies. However, if our brains release these hormones too often it is bad for our health. People who are stressed for a long time may be more likely to get colds, heart disease, and other health problems. This is why it is so important to learn how to change your thoughts that cause negative feelings.

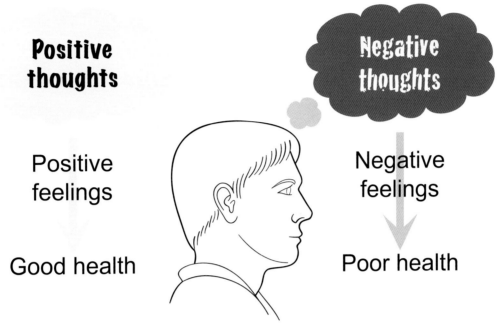

Thought Errors

Sometimes people get in the habit of having thoughts that are not helpful. Thoughts that are not helpful or unhealthy are called "thought errors." You may feel bad or get upset out of habit and find out later that the reason you got upset was your own "thought error."[11]

All people make thought errors from time to time. Many people make thought errors that cause them to feel sad or upset. If you are aware of the most common thought errors, you can catch yourself and correct your thinking. Read the list of thought errors below. Think about which ones are familiar to you.[11] Remember: thought errors are very common.

"Thought Errors"

Twelve Common Thought Errors:

1 **All-or-nothing thinking:** When you see things in only two categories such as black or white.

   Example: You see yourself as a failure if you are not perfect.

   Example: "Nothing I ever do is right."

   Tinnitus example: "If my tinnitus is loud when I wake up in the morning I know I will have a bad day."

   Corrected thought: "I'm learning ways to have a good day even when my tinnitus is loud."

   My example: _____

2 **Over-simplifying:** When you see one bad event as a pattern that never changes.

   Example: You get on the wrong train one time and think, "I'll never learn how to use the subway."

   Tinnitus example: "I was awake all night from my tinnitus. This will happen every night."

   Corrected thought: "Last night my tinnitus kept me awake, but most nights I eventually fall asleep."

   My example: _____

3 **Focusing on wrong details:** When you pick out a single detail and focus on it. You don't think about other more positive details.

   Example: "I got a 60% on my math homework. I'm a terrible student."

   Tinnitus example: "My tinnitus made it hard to enjoy dinner with a friend."

   Corrected thought: "My tinnitus was really loud at dinner. However, it was great to see my friend again and to catch up."

   My example: _____

4   **Jumping to conclusions:** When you think an event was unpleasant even though there are no facts to support that. You might assume that you know what someone else is thinking or assume things will turn out badly.

Example: "If I go to the party then I won't know anyone and will not have fun."

Tinnitus example: "My tinnitus kept me awake last night. The next day I met a friend for coffee. I was really tired and didn't talk much. I'll bet he thought I was boring."

Corrected thought: "It was difficult to be so tired all day. I told my friend about my tinnitus keeping me awake. He was very supportive."

My example: _____

5   **Over-estimating:** When you think things are more important than they really are (such as your goof-up or someone else's success).

Example: "She turned me down when I asked her to go on a date with me. I don't know how to talk to women. I'll be alone forever."

Tinnitus example: "My tinnitus makes me moody. No one wants to be around me."

Corrected thought: "Sometimes I'm moody and other times I am in a great mood. I have friends who know me and understand me."

My example: _____

6   **Under-estimating:** When you think things are less important than they really are (such as your success or someone else's faults).

Example: "I know I got a 95% on the test but I could have done better."

Tinnitus example: "I know I learned how to get to sleep even though my tinnitus is loud. I also started using soothing sound for my tinnitus at work. Even so, I'll never learn to deal with my tinnitus."

Corrected thought: "I can deal with my tinnitus by making small changes. It may not be gone, but I don't notice my tinnitus as often."

My example: _____

7   Assuming the worst: When you think something is much worse than it really is.

Example: A woman who got a low grade on a quiz thinks it's the end of her college career."

Tinnitus example: "I'm going to become deaf from my tinnitus."

Corrected thought: "My doctor said tinnitus won't make me deaf. It just feels strange to hear this ringing in my ears all the time and not know why."

My example: _____

8   Emotional thoughts: When you think that your emotions show the way things really are. You might think, "I feel it, so it must be true."

Example: "I feel like I'm the only one who cleans up around here so you must not be helping."

Tinnitus example: "I feel like no one knows what I am going through with my tinnitus. I feel all alone."

Corrected thought: "People know what I am going through when I explain tinnitus to them.

My example: _____

9   "Should" statements: When you say "should" and "shouldn't" to try to get yourself to do hard tasks. These statements tend to make you feel guilty. Also included are statements with the words "must" and "ought."

Example: "I should eat healthier and stop eating food I like."

Tinnitus example: "I should not have to deal with tinnitus during the best years of my life."

Corrected thought: "Tinnitus isn't what I expected when I retired, but I can deal with it."

My example: _____

10   Labeling: Attaching a bad label to yourself or others.

Example: "He lost his keys so he's stupid."

Tinnitus example: "I can't deal with my tinnitus so I'm a weak person."

Corrected thought: "Sometimes it's hard to deal with my tinnitus. I do my best to stay healthy and active. I practice methods for managing my reactions to tinnitus from the workbook. However, sometimes the tinnitus still bothers me. That is normal."

My example: _____

11   Making Things Personal: You see yourself as the cause of some negative event when you are not responsible. You ignore other details.

Example: "My doctor was not nice to me because I was sick."

Tinnitus example: "My tinnitus made it hard for me to enjoy the picnic. I caused everyone else to have a bad time, too."

Corrected thought: "My tinnitus made it hard for me to enjoy the picnic. No one can have fun all of the time."

My example: _____

12   Blaming: You blame others for your problems. You may also blame yourself for other people's problems.

Example: "I didn't get the job because you didn't call to give me a pep-talk before my meeting."

Tinnitus example: "My tinnitus wouldn't be a problem if my wife was more supportive."

Corrected thought: "It would be helpful if my wife was more supportive. Either way I would have to work at dealing with my tinnitus."

My example: _____

Correcting Thought Errors

So how can you control negative feelings? Your thoughts determine the feelings you experience. You may not be able to change events, or tinnitus. However, the way you think about an event *is under your control.* Change your thoughts, and your feelings will change too. Next you will learn a step-by-step approach to changing thoughts.

Changing Thoughts - Step-by-Step:

Please use the Changing Thoughts Exercise form on p. 56 to complete the steps below.

Step 1: Event. Identify what was going on when you started feeling bad - what happened? Sometimes it is hard to remember the event that was happening that made you feel bad until later. If this is the case for you, go to the second step and come back to this step later.

Step 2: Thoughts. Now try to write down a thought you had just before you started feeling bad or upset. What was the first thought that came into your mind? You may have had many thoughts just before you started feeling bad. If you had more than one thought, pick the one that made you feel the worst.

Step 3: Feelings. Write down any bad or upsetting feelings you are having. For example, sad, angry, jealous, or disappointed.

Step 4: Evidence *for.* Examine the thought you described in Step 2. Write down evidence that this statement is true where it says "Evidence For" below. Our thoughts often have some truth to them, but some have many more errors. Write down what is true about the thought in the "Evidence For" box.

Step 5: Evidence *against.* Again, examine the thought you described in Step 2. Identify evidence that this statement is not true. In the next box where it says "Evidence Against" write down reasons the thought may *not* be true. Can you identify any of the 12 thought errors from the list? (You can have more than one thought error in one thought.)

Step 6: New positive thought. Write down a new thought about the event that is more helpful. This step requires a lot of practice. With practice it will become more natural to create new positive thoughts. Sometimes it helps to say statements that apply to many things. For example, "I am whole and complete," or "I love and accept myself."

New positive thoughts should be:

- *brief*
- *easy to remember*
- *thoughts you believe are true*
- *thoughts that apply to your life*
- *helpful*

Step 7: Feelings when you think the new thought. As you practice, pay attention to how you feel when you have positive thoughts instead of negative thoughts. Do you notice your tinnitus as much? Are your muscles relaxed?

Step 8: Picture yourself in the future. Look at the negative thought from Step 1 again. Think of a time in the future when you might have that thought again. Picture yourself thinking the positive thought from Step 6 instead.

Changing Thoughts Exercise

Directions: Keep track of three situations when you felt bad or upset during the week. Practice changing your thoughts in each situation using these steps.

Steps	Example	Your situation 1	Your situation 2	Your situation 3
Step 1: Event	My tinnitus isn't getting any better			
Step 2: Thoughts	Why can't anyone help me?			
Step 3: Feelings	Helpless, frustrated and angry			
Step 4: Evidence for	I've been to so many doctors and still have tinnitus			
Step 5: Evidence against	I fell asleep easily last night. Maybe using sound is helping me, even if my tinnitus isn't any quieter.			
Step 6: New positive thought	I probably can't make my tinnitus quieter. Even so, I can find ways to feel better even if the tinnitus doesn't change.			
Step 7: Feelings when you think the new thought	Happier, more confident			

Step 8: Picture yourself in the future. Think of an event in the future when you might have the negative thoughts again. Picture yourself thinking the positive thought instead.

56

The Changing Thoughts and Feelings Worksheet

Next you will learn about the Changing Thoughts and Feelings Worksheet. You will use this Worksheet to develop a "plan of action" to change your thoughts and feelings about tinnitus. You learned three skills in this section (Part 3): (1) relaxation exercises; (2) pleasant activity scheduling; and (3) changing thoughts. You will be able to choose from these three skills when you make your "plan of action."

Blank Changing Thoughts and Feelings Worksheets are in the back of this workbook. They are on the back side of the Sound Plan Worksheets. Steps for completing the Changing Thoughts and Feelings Worksheet are listed below. There is an example of a completed Worksheet on page 59. The example Worksheet was completed for "Joe." "Joe" is described on page 60.

Steps for Completing the Worksheet

1 Use the Tinnitus Problem Checklist (p. 29) to list situations when your tinnitus is most bothersome.

2 For each situation that you list, use a separate Changing Thoughts and Feelings Worksheet.

    a Write the situation at the top of the Worksheet (#1)

    b Decide which of the three skills you will use to manage this situation (#2 on the Worksheet)

    c Write down the details for each skill you will use (#3)

    d Write down how you feel after doing the exercise (#4)

3 Try each skill you chose at least three times over the next week (#4 on the Worksheet).

4 Rate how helpful each trial was (#4).

5 At any time, write down what works and what doesn't work (#5).

Ongoing Use of the Worksheet

It takes trial and error to learn what works best in each situation. Use the Worksheet on a regular basis to change and improve your action plans. Also, use the Worksheet to create new plans for different situations. Learning to change your thoughts and feelings takes time and practice. If the exercises don't help right away, keep practicing. They can become more useful over time.

Changing Thoughts and Feelings Worksheet

Joe

1. From the Tinnitus Problem Checklist, write down one bothersome tinnitus situation *My tinnitus makes it hard for me to concentrate at work*

2. Check one or more of the three skills to manage the situation

☑ **Relaxation exercises**

breathe	
Relax	
imagine	

☑ **Plan pleasant activities**

golf, write, walk	
Pleasant activities	
dance, paint	

☑ **Changing thoughts**

Think → Feel

3. Write down the details for each skill you will use

Relaxation exercises
- ☑ *Deep breathing*
- ☑ *Imagery*
- ☑ *Other* *meditation*

Plan pleasant activities
- Activity 1 *take a walk during lunch*
- Activity 2 _____
- Activity 3 _____

Changing thoughts
- Old thought *I can't think about anything but my tinnitus*
- New thought *There are many ways I can focus on things other than my tinnitus*

EXAMPLE

4. Use your plan over the next week. How helpful was each exercise?

Not at all / A little / Moderately / Very much / Extremely

Relaxation exercises: ☑ Moderately

Plan pleasant activities: ☑ Moderately; ☑ Very much

Changing thoughts: ☑ A little

5. Comments
When you find something that works well (or not so well) please comment. You do not need to wait 1 week to write your comments.

This helps!
This helps a little
This feels good

It was easier for me to concentrate after taking a walk

I feel better

Changing Thoughts and Feelings Example: "Joe"

Joe works in an office on a computer all day. Because of his tinnitus, it is hard for him to concentrate on his work. Using the Sound Plan Worksheet, Joe found that keeping his radio on helped him to notice his tinnitus less. The radio is all he needs to help him concentrate during normal work days. However, when he is really stressed he still has a hard time concentrating.

Joe now takes a break when he feels very stressed and cannot concentrate. He practices imagery for 10 minutes and then goes back to working. Practicing imagery helps Joe get his mind completely off of his tinnitus for a short time. That helps him relax. Once he is relaxed it is much easier for him to concentrate on his work.

When Joe is especially frustrated, he tries to identify an event that made him feel that way. He then identifies thoughts he is having about the event. He writes down more positive thoughts and keeps them on a post-it note on his computer. This helps Joe have more realistic and helpful thoughts. As a result, he feels less frustration and stress.

Joe enjoys walking. He now takes a walk during his lunch. This pleasant activity helps Joe get his mind off of his tinnitus.

Summary

In this section (Part 3) you learned things you can do (skills) to change your reactions to tinnitus and to feel better. They are Relaxation Exercises, Pleasant Activity Scheduling, and Changing Thoughts. In Part 2 you learned about using sound in different ways to manage your reactions to tinnitus. Experiment with all of the ideas that you learned about in Parts 2 and 3. As you experiment you will get better at managing your tinnitus. You also will learn which ideas work best for you.

Some people may need more help dealing with their tinnitus and other problems. Contact a mental health provider right away if you feel very sad or worried. A mental health provider can talk to you about your tinnitus or any other problem. This provider can help you find more ways to deal with your tinnitus and problems in your life.

If you want to hurt yourself or are suicidal, go to your local emergency room immediately or call the **National Suicide Prevention Hotline toll free: 1-800-273-TALK or 1-800-273-8255**.

Part 4. Protect Your Ears!

In Part 1 we explained that we cannot change the tinnitus. But, we can change our *reactions* to it. Parts 2 and 3 gave step-by-step instructions to learn how to manage reactions to tinnitus. Part 4 focuses on protecting your ears from very loud sound.

Loud noise can cause hearing loss and tinnitus. If you already have hearing loss or tinnitus, loud noise can cause *more* damage and *make the tinnitus worse.* The louder a sound is, the faster it can damage your hearing (see figure on next page). Power tools, lawnmowers, and chain saws are very loud. You should never use them without hearing protection (earplugs and/or earmuffs). Loud music, whether live or recorded, can cause damage. (If you listen to music for your tinnitus, you should always play the music at soft levels.) Even traffic noise can cause damage if you are exposed to it for many hours in one day. Driving with the window open for several hours at a time can cause noise damage, especially in the ear by the window.

You should always wear hearing protection when you are around loud noise. You need to find hearing protection that is handy and easy to use. There are many different types of earplugs and earmuffs. You can get them from:

- hearing specialists
- sporting goods stores
- industrial supply sources
- home improvement stores
- websites on the internet (see Appendix J)

The Louder a Sound is,
the Faster it Can Damage Your Hearing

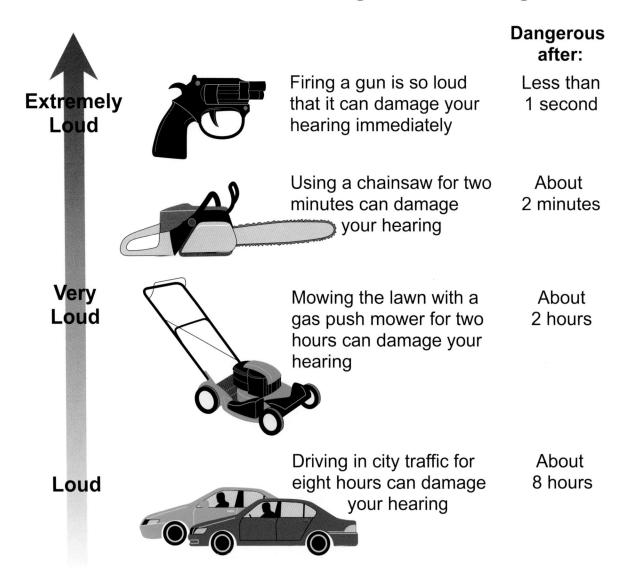

Dangerous after:

Extremely Loud — Firing a gun is so loud that it can damage your hearing immediately — Less than 1 second

Using a chainsaw for two minutes can damage your hearing — About 2 minutes

Very Loud — Mowing the lawn with a gas push mower for two hours can damage your hearing — About 2 hours

Loud — Driving in city traffic for eight hours can damage your hearing — About 8 hours

Standard Earplugs

Standard (non-custom) earplugs are low cost and "one size fits all." Yellow foam earplugs are the most common. All earplugs can protect against loud noise but they must be used properly. Foam earplugs need to be inserted almost completely into the ear canal (with very little of the plug left outside of the canal - see the photo below). If they are not used properly, then they might not give you enough protection from sound. You can try different earplugs to find what works best for you. Some dealers offer "trial packs" with a variety of earplugs.

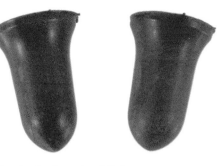

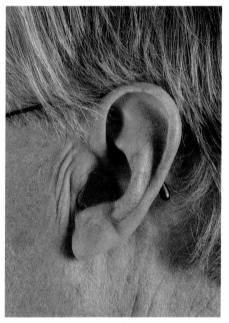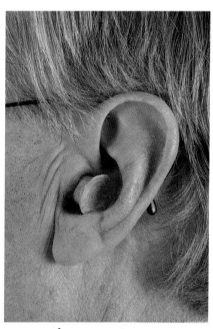

correct use   **incorrect use**

Custom Earplugs

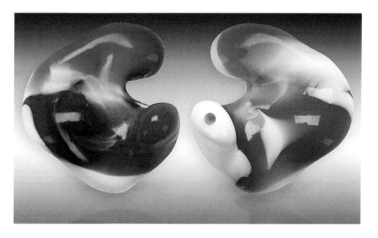

Custom earplugs are custom molded to the ears. An audiologist can have them made for you. Custom earplugs usually are very comfortable, easy to use, and can be used for years.

Photo of custom earplugs courtesy of E.A.R., Inc.

Hi-fi Earplugs

"Hi-fi" earplugs reduce loudness equally for both low and high pitches. This avoids the muffled effect that is caused by most earplugs. Hi-fi earplugs were designed for musicians who need to hear music clearly. These

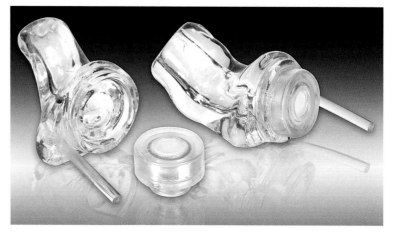

earplugs also work well when you need to hear speech in a noisy environment.

Electronic Earplugs

Electronic earplugs allow you to hear soft sounds, but very loud sounds, like gunshots, are reduced. These earplugs are used mainly by hunters. Non-electronic earplugs also are available for this purpose.

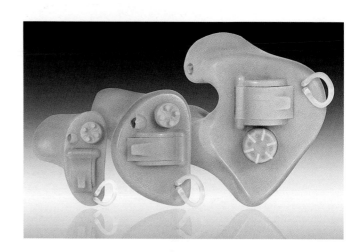

Earmuffs

Earmuffs can be used *instead of* earplugs or *along with* earplugs. Earmuffs should be worn along with earplugs when you are around extremely loud noise like gun fire or chainsaws. It is important that earmuffs fit snugly around the ears to get a good seal. Wearing glasses or a hood under the earmuffs will cause them to be less effective.

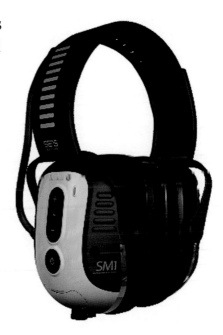

All photos on this page courtesy of E.A.R., Inc.

APPENDIX A
Description of Tinnitus

How is "Tinnitus" Pronounced?

What is the right way to say "tinnitus"? This question is often debated and not even all dictionaries agree. It has been pronounced tin-EYE-tus and TIN-uh-tus. Either way you say it is fine.

What is Tinnitus?

Sound vibrations in the air become coded signals that the brain interprets as sound. With tinnitus, there are no sound wave vibrations causing nerve fibers to fire. With most forms of tinnitus, some of the nerve fibers are firing on their own. The brain interprets these signals as sound.

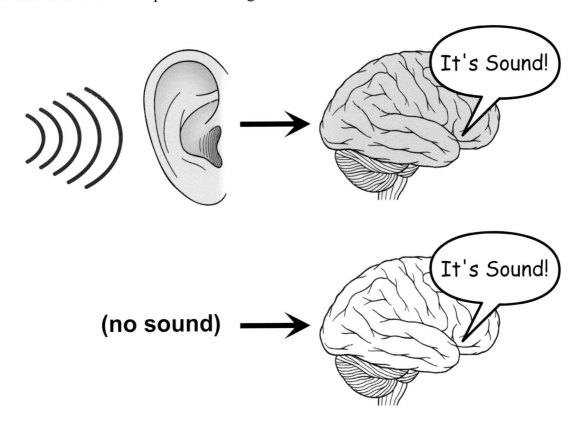

Does Everyone's Tinnitus Sound the Same?

Just about every type of sound has been reported when patients have been asked to describe the sound of their tinnitus. "Ringing" and "high pitched tone" are reported most often. Other sounds commonly reported include "hissing," "high tension wire," "buzzing," "sizzling," and "crickets." Many people hear more than one sound.

How Many People Have Tinnitus?

Studies show that about 10 to 15 percent of all adults have permanent tinnitus. The American Tinnitus Association reports that about 50 million Americans have tinnitus. Most people with tinnitus are not bothered by it. Some people have tinnitus that is very bothersome.

(This appendix adapted from Henry, Zaugg, & Schechter, Clinical guide for audiologic tinnitus management II: Treatment. American Journal of Audiology, 14:49-70, 2005)

APPENDIX B
What Causes Tinnitus?

We don't know what causes tinnitus, but we have insights based on what is known about the hearing system. You will now learn how sound is detected by the ear and processed by the brain. This will help you understand what might be going on in the brain when tinnitus is present.

The "Microphone" Part of the Ear

The three major parts of the ear are the outer ear, middle ear, and inner ear. The inner ear includes the cochlea, a fluid-filled bony structure that is shaped like a snail shell. It is smaller than the tip of your little finger but very complex. The cochlea performs a task like that of a microphone. That is, the cochlea converts sound wave vibrations into electrical signals. These electrical signals are transmitted by nerves into the brain.

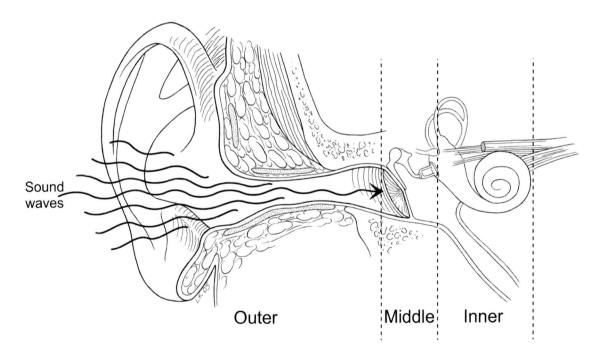

Adapted with permission from Henry JA, Trune DR, Robb MJA, Jastreboff PJ. Tinnitus Retraining Therapy: Patient Counseling Guide. San Diego: Plural Publishing, Inc.; 2007.

Hair Cells

Inside the cochlea is a "ribbon" of tiny cells called "hair cells" that change sound vibrations into nerve signals. They are called "hair cells" because each cell has up to 150 "hairs" projecting from the top. The hair cells are laid out on the "ribbon" like keys on a piano keyboard. These hair cells cannot be seen by the human eye and need to magnified by a powerful electron microscope to be seen. Hair cells are even "tuned" like keys on a keyboard, from low pitches at one end to high pitches at the other. Sound vibrations travel to the hair cells through the fluid in the cochlea. The vibrations in the fluid cause the hairs to vibrate. Each pitch (or "frequency") of sound triggers hair cells that are tuned to that frequency. There are about 16,000 hair cells that are lined up - in three rows of outer hair cells and one row of inner hair cells. The inner and outer hair cells serve different purposes, and damage to each type causes different problems.

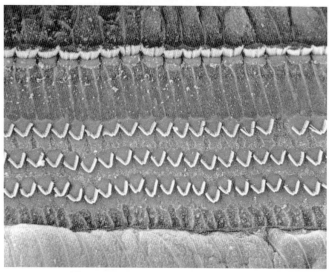

Inner hair cells

Outer hair cells

Photo courtesy of David J. Lim, MD,
House Ear Institute, Los Angeles, CA.

Outer hair cells

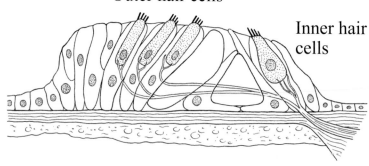

Inner hair cells

Auditory (Hearing) Nerve Sends Nerve Impulses Into the Brain

The hearing nerve connects the hair cells in the cochlea to the brain. The hearing nerve is like an electric cable. It is one and a half inches long. It contains thousands of individual "wires" (nerve fibers). Our hearing information enters the brain through the auditory nerve just like all of the information from a microphone travels through a cable.

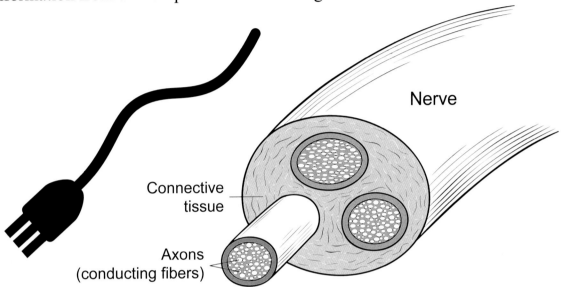

Adapted with permission from Henry JA, Trune DR, Robb MJA, Jastreboff PJ. Tinnitus Retraining Therapy: Patient Counseling Guide. San Diego: Plural Publishing, Inc.; 2007.

What is a "Nerve Impulse"?

The hearing system, from the hearing nerve up through the brain, consists entirely of nerve fibers. When a hair cell is triggered by a vibration, nerve fibers connected to the hair cell discharge. This is like firing a gun. Nerve fibers have one task to perform: to send impulses from one end to the other.

How do we "Hear" Nerve Impulses?

The brain works kind of like a computer. Computer language is based on zeros and ones. A single zero doesn't mean anything and a single one doesn't mean anything. It is the *patterns* of zeros and ones that are meaningful to a computer. In the same way, the brain recognizes patterns of on-and-off discharges of nerve fibers.

The fibers in the hearing nerve are like wires in a telephone cable. Each wire can transmit information independent of the other wires. The brain is able to "read" the information coming in from all of the fibers at the same time. A cross section of the hearing nerve will, at any point in time, reveal a pattern of some fibers firing and some not firing. The brain "takes a picture" of this patterned activity thousands of times every second. Between each picture the pattern changes. The brain is able to interpret these coded patterns as they stream in from the hearing nerve. This results in the perception of sound.

Final Destination of Nerve Impulses: Cortex

The outer layer of the brain is the "cerebral cortex." This is where all conscious perception (including listening) takes place. Signals that travel up the hearing pathways encounter "relay stations" on their way up to the cortex. The nerve fibers branch at each higher level. There are about 30,000 fibers in the hearing nerve that branch as soon as they enter the brainstem. They eventually branch into about 10,000,000 fibers. The brain continually processes coded information contained within all of these fibers. The end result is the conscious perception of sounds that occur outside of the body.

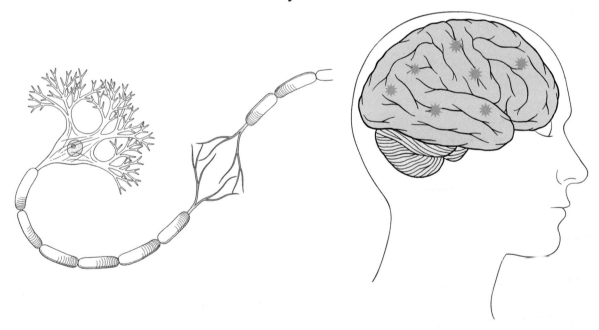

Adapted with permission from Henry JA, Trune DR, Robb MJA, Jastreboff PJ. Tinnitus Retraining Therapy: Patient Counseling Guide. San Diego: Plural Publishing, Inc.; 2007.

What Causes Tinnitus?

We don't know what causes the pattern of nerve discharges that our brain perceives as tinnitus. We know that certain events such as loud noises damage hair cells in the inner ear. This can result in hearing loss and/or tinnitus. It can be assumed that regions of damaged hair cells are involved in the making of tinnitus. Removing "abnormal hair cell activity" from entering the brain should logically "turn off" a person's tinnitus. Some patients had one of their hearing nerves severed to try and cut off the source of their tinnitus. All of these patients became deaf on that side, and the tinnitus returned for most of them. This suggests that the source of tinnitus can be anywhere within the hearing nervous system of the brain.

Reported Causes of Tinnitus

Many people don't know what caused their tinnitus. When a cause is reported, *loud noise* is blamed most often. Other causes include:

- *Trauma to the head or neck* (whiplash, concussion, skull fracture, etc.)

- *Ear conditions* (excessive ear wax, infection, inflammation, Meniere's disease, otosclerosis, presbycusis, acoustic tumor, etc.)

- *Other reported causes* (heart problems, strokes, thyroid disease, drugs, surgery, stress, diabetes, multiple sclerosis, and TMJ disorder, etc.)

(This appendix adapted from Henry, Zaugg, & Schechter, Clinical guide for audiologic tinnitus management II: Treatment. American Journal of Audiology, 14:49-70, 2005)

APPENDIX C
Methods of Tinnitus Management

Two Approaches to Tinnitus Management

There are two overall approaches to tinnitus management:

1. Eliminate tinnitus or reduce its loudness

2. Reduce the person's reactions to the tinnitus

First Approach: Eliminate Tinnitus or Reduce its Loudness

Prescription Drugs

Many drugs have been used for tinnitus. These are drugs designed to manage other problems such as depression, anxiety, or lack of sleep. Drugs can occasionally reduce the loudness of tinnitus. Choosing a drug for this purpose is a trial-and-error process. Using any drug to treat tinnitus must be approached with great care because of the potential for side effects. Their use can be habit forming or even addictive. Some drugs, and mixes of drugs, can make a person's tinnitus louder.[12]

Surgery

Most tinnitus is the sensorineural (nerve) type for which surgery is not an option.[13] In rare cases, tinnitus can be caused by:

- muscular spasms,

- blood vessel constriction,

- metabolic conditions, or

- some other source of noise in the body.

These kinds of sounds have been referred to as "somatosounds" or "objective tinnitus." Some doctors are skilled in diagnosing this, and surgery can sometimes help treat the cause.[14] The hearing nerve was cut for some patients totry and cut off the source of the tinnitus. This is not done anymore because these patients became deaf in that ear, and the tinnitus often returned. Another rare cause of tinnitus is a (often benign) tumor on the hearing nerve. When this occurs, the tinnitus usually is in one ear. It appears slowly along with hearing loss in the same ear. Such tumors can be removed with surgery.

Electrical Stimulation

Some studies have described the use of electrical stimulation to reduce the loudness of tinnitus. This involves applying a small electric current to some area around the ears. This has been known to help some patients. No one yet can consistently achieve this effect.[15] Some patients with *cochlear implants* report that their tinnitus is reduced when the implant is activated. A cochlear implant requires surgery that involves threading a wire through the cochlea. The wire contains tiny electrodes that produce electrical signals that activate nerve endings in the cochlea. This surgery usually is not an option for tinnitus patients unless they have no usable hearing in both ears.

Transcranial Magnetic Stimulation

Transcranial magnetic stimulation (TMS) is a new method that may suppress tinnitus in some people.[16-18] An electromagnetic coil is held against the head over the region of interest.[17] Passing current through the coil causes a magnetic field to pass through the cortex (outer layer of the brain). Oscillating the strength of the current (called repetitive TMS, or rTMS) causes the magnetic field to fluctuate. Low-frequency rTMS decreases cortical excitability and sensory perception. High-frequency rTMS increases excitability. Studies have shown that low-frequency rTMS can help with disorders that are linked with increased cortical activity. This finding led to studies looking at its ability to suppress tinnitus. These studies are "promising," but further research is needed.

Use of Sound

In Part 2 of this workbook we describe how to use sound to *manage reactions* to tinnitus. Sound cannot "eliminate tinnitus or reduce its loudness." However, sound can give the *perception* that the tinnitus is eliminated or reduced in loudness. For example, patients treated with Tinnitus Masking usually are fitted with masking devices that fit in or over the ears. The devices present wide-band noise (sounds like "shhh") to the ears. The noise can cover, or "mask," the tinnitus. Masking the tinnitus gives the *perception* that the tinnitus has been eliminated. Even if the tinnitus is not completely masked, hearing the noise can give the perception that the tinnitus is reduced in loudness.

Does the "First Approach" Work?

Anyone with tinnitus wants the sound eliminated. They want a "cure," which is the main goal of the "first approach." If the main goal can't be met, then the "first approach" tries to at least reduce the loudness of tinnitus. To date, there is no safe, consistent way to eliminate tinnitus or to reduce its loudness for most patients. Using sound can give the *perception* that the tinnitus is gone or reduced in loudness. However, another sound must be presented to the ear to cause this perception.

Second Approach: Reduce Reactions to Tinnitus

Most therapies for tinnitus do not try to eliminate tinnitus or reduce its loudness. Rather, they try to reduce the person's *reactions* to the tinnitus. This is what is meant by tinnitus *management*. There are many methods that are used to manage tinnitus.

Prescription Drugs

As described above, drugs often are used in the attempt to eliminate tinnitus or reduce its loudness ("first approach"). Drugs also are used to reduce *emotional reactions* to tinnitus. Prescription drugs can reduce reactions to tinnitus by:

- calming anxieties,

- elevating mood,

- relieving depression, and/or

- inducing sleep.[19]

If your reaction to tinnitus involves anxiety, an anti-anxiety drug may help. If you have trouble sleeping because of the tinnitus, drugs can restore restful sleep. If you have depression, treatment of it may lessen the severity of the tinnitus problem. *However*, regular use of drugs to treat tinnitus can cause side effects and/or addiction to the drugs. See your medical doctor if you are depressed, stressed, anxious, or have trouble sleeping.

Psychological Approaches

Many psychological approaches have been used to manage tinnitus. These include, but are not limited to, the following.

- *Relaxation training* involves deep breathing, imagery, and other exercises intended to reduce stress. The goal is to reduce overall reactions to stress and/or provide a distraction from tinnitus. If tinnitus causes stress, relaxation training can reduce the stress. Relaxation training requires concentration and practice to be used effectively.

- *Cognitive therapy* (also called "cognitive restructuring") involves helping people change how they think about their tinnitus to help them feel better.

- *Cognitive-Behavioral Therapy (CBT)* combines cognitive therapy with everyday activity changes. CBT originally was used to treat people with depression, anxiety, and chronic pain.[20] CBT was adapted for use with people who have tinnitus, and became the main psychological approach to managing tinnitus.[5] The method normally requires about eight sessions. It is conducted weekly in either a group or one-on-one setting. The goal is to reduce reactions to tinnitus and stress associated with tinnitus. A self-management guide using principles of CBT has been published.[6] Part 3 of this workbook is based on the use of CBT for tinnitus.

Sound-based Methods

Some methods of tinnitus management rely on the use of sound. These are the main methods used by audiologists. Each of these methods uses sound in different ways.[9]

Hearing Aids

Before we talk about the different sound-based methods, we first need to mention that hearing aids often are helpful for tinnitus. Many patients who have hearing loss and tinnitus discover that hearing aids alone are all they need to successfully manage their reactions to tinnitus.

Hearing aids can be helpful in managing reactions to tinnitus because they:
- Increase **background** sound (reduces contrast between tinnitus and quiet environments)

- Make it easier to hear **soothing** sounds (to reduce stress caused by tinnitus)

- Make it easier to hear **interesting** sounds (to help shift attention away from tinnitus)

- Make difficult listening situations less stressful

Tinnitus Masking (TM)

As described above, using sound with TM can give the *perception* that tinnitus is eliminated or reduced in loudness. However, the main goal of TM is to use sound to provide a sense of relief.[21,22] Patients normally are fitted with ear-level devices that present wide-band noise (a "shhh" sound) to the ears. Patients are instructed to adjust the noise to the level that provides the greatest sense of relief. Patients also are advised to use all kinds of sound-producing devices to achieve relief. These devices include CDs, tabletop fountains, sound machines, sound pillows, etc.[1] Counseling also is used with Masking, but the use of sound is the primary mode of management.[21]

• **The use of sound with TM is an example of using *environmental sound as soothing sound***

	Environmental	Music	Speech
Soothing	✓		
Background			
Interesting			

Tinnitus Retraining Therapy (TRT)

The method of TRT has two basic components: educational counseling and sound therapy.[2, 23] Educational counseling is designed to remove any fears linked with the tinnitus. The counseling is like a class. The clinician is the "teacher." Detailed lectures about the "neurophysiological model" are taught.[24] For sound therapy, patients are told to "enrich their sound environment" at all times with soft, pleasant background sound. For those who are most severely bothered by their tinnitus, ear-level devices are advised for use each day for at least one year. Patients with less severe tinnitus normally do not use ear-level devices.[25, 26]

Unlike Tinnitus Masking, the use of sound with TRT is not meant to give a sense of relief. With TRT, the patient should hear the tinnitus clearly, but with constant sound in the background. The constant sound reduces the contrast between the tinnitus and the quiet environment. Patients are supposed to use sound in this way everyday to eventually achieve "habituation." Habituation for TRT means that you stop reacting to the tinnitus and stop noticing it is there.

- **The use of sound with TRT is an example of using *environmental sound as background sound.***

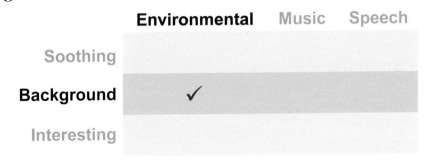

Neuromonics Tinnitus Treatment (NTT)
[Note: Any discussion about Neuromonics refers to the company Neuromonics Pty Ltd. The company promotes and supports their method. The VA does not endorse Neuromonics at this time. Any information provided about Neuromonics is for information purposes only.] NTT is different from the other forms of sound-based tinnitus management in that providers must work with a company to receive all training, materials, wearable devices, and support. Neuromonics Pty Ltd is a company based in Australia with operations also in the United States. NTT previously was referred to as acoustic desensitization therapy.[27]

NTT patients use a wearable listening device 2-3 hours per day for at least 6 months.[3] The device is a like an MP3 player, and plays Baroque and New Age music. For each patient, the device is customized by the company so that the sound is adjusted ("equalized") for any hearing loss. During the first 2 months of treatment (stage 1) wide-band noise (described as "shower sound") is added to the music. Patients are instructed to achieve a "high level of interaction" between the music and their tinnitus. The objective of stage 1 is to attain a "sense of relief and control over the tinnitus, and promote a reduction in general anxiety levels" (p. 149).[3]

- **The use of sound during stage 1 of NTT is an example of *using a combination of music and environmental sound as soothing sound.***

	Environmental	**Music**	Speech
Soothing	✓	✓	
Background			
Interesting			

During the next 4 months (stage 2) the noise is removed. Patients are instructed to gradually reduce the volume of the music to decrease the level of interaction between the music and the tinnitus. The objective of stage 2 is essentially the same as for TRT: less awareness of, and less reaction to, the tinnitus. The company has conducted its own clinical studies. No independent, controlled studies have been done to evaluate NTT.

- **The use of sound during stage 2 of NTT is an example of *using music as soothing sound*, transitioning to *using music as background sound.***

	Environmental	**Music**	Speech
Soothing		✓	
Background		✓	
Interesting			

Progressive Tinnitus Management (PTM)
PTM is the method that is described in this workbook.[7] A unique aspect of PTM is that sound can be used in different ways for different situations when tinnitus is a problem. PTM describes three types of sound to manage reactions to tinnitus:

1 Soothing sound
2 Background sound
3 Interesting sound

Different situations when tinnitus is a problem require different approaches. PTM involves using the Sound Plan Worksheet (p. 30) to decide how to use sound for each tinnitus-problem situation. For each type of sound (soothing, background, interesting), you can use environmental sound, music, or speech. Depending on the situation, a different combination is most appropriate. This all has been described in Part 2 of this workbook. Additional details about PTM, including assessment procedures, specific counseling information, and the use of hearing aids, have been published.[8, 9, 28]

- **The use of sound with PTM can involve all combinations of *types* of sound (soothing, background, interesting) and environmental sound, music, and speech.**

	Environmental	Music	Speech
Soothing	✓	✓	✓
Background	✓	✓	✓
Interesting	✓	✓	✓

PTM is not limited to using sound. As described in Part 3 of this workbook, different components of Cognitive-Behavioral Therapy (CBT) are also used. Using sound alone may not be enough for some people. It may also be important to address cognitive and emotional aspects of tinnitus. CBT provides a good framework for addressing those concerns.

"Complementary and Alternative" Methods
There are many tinnitus treatments considered "complementary and alternative." These include but are not limited to:

- nutritional supplements,
- homeopathic remedies,
- acupuncture,
- naturopathic medicine,
- hypnosis

Many people are convinced that the herb gingko biloba is useful. Large-scale controlled studies have shown no helpful effect of gingko.[29] There are nutritional remedies that may include "tinnitus" in their name. These are mixtures of herbs and vitamins. They often include zinc, ginkgo, and/or vitamin B-12. Many claims have been made. There is no scientific proof that any of these remedies are effective, other than for isolated cases.[30]

(Portions of this appendix adapted from Henry, Zaugg, & Schechter, Clinical guide for audiologic tinnitus management II: Treatment. American Journal of Audiology, 14:49-70, 2005)

APPENDIX D
What To Do When Everyday Sounds Are Too Loud (not related to using hearing aids)

*Bill Smith is bothered by **everyday sounds**. (This problem is sometimes called **hyperacusis**.) Kitchen sounds and the vacuum cleaner are too loud for him. He is bothered by road noise when he drives. It seems like everything at church is too loud. What should Bill do? Believe it or not, being around more sound can make things **better**! And, staying away from sound can make his problem **worse**! What??? He should add **more** sound??? Keep reading and we'll explain . . .*

There are three things you can do if everyday sounds are too loud for you.

1 Keep yourself surrounded with sound that is comfortable for you

2 Listen to sounds that you enjoy as often as you can

3 Only wear hearing protection when you really need to

I. Keep yourself surrounded with sound that is comfortable for you.

Why should I keep myself surrounded with sound? Let's start by thinking about your eyes and how they adjust to light. Imagine sitting in a dark movie theater and then going outside into the daylight. Everything seems brighter to you than it does to people who were not sitting in the dark. Your eyes had adjusted to the dark and now they have to readjust to the daylight.

Your ears adjust to sound kind of like your eyes adjust to light. If you stay away from sound, your ears will slowly adjust to the quiet. After a while, everyday sounds will seem louder and harder to tolerate. Avoiding sound will only make the problem worse.

If you keep yourself surrounded with sound, your ears will readjust. It will slowly become easier for you to tolerate everyday sounds. You should only use sounds that are comfortable for you. It usually takes at least a few weeks of being around sound for this change to happen.

How do I keep myself surrounded with sound? You can use any sound that is not annoying. (The sound can be either neutral or pleasant.) Here are some ideas:

- listen to music at a comfortable level
- listen to radio shows
- play recordings of nature sounds
- keep a fan running
- use a tabletop water fountain

Another choice: Some people wear small instruments in their ears that make a "shhh" sound. These instruments are called *in-the-ear noise generators* or *maskers*. Your audiologist can tell you more about them.

2. Listen to sounds that you enjoy as often as you can.

Why should I listen to sounds that I enjoy as often as I can? We just talked about the problem of everyday sounds being too loud (*hyperacusis*). Many people also have another problem. They just *don't like* certain sounds, but *not because they are too loud*. (This problem is sometimes called *misophonia*.) If you don't like certain sounds, you should make a point of listening to sounds that you enjoy. Spending time enjoying sound can help you get better at tolerating everyday sounds that you don't like.

3. Only wear hearing protection when you really need to.

Why should I use ear protection *only* when I really need to? When everyday sounds seem too loud, some people start using ear protection all the time. Remember that avoiding sound will make the problem worse. Only use ear protection when sounds are dangerously loud or uncomfortably loud. *As soon* as the sound around you is at a safe and comfortable level, take the ear protection off. The goal is to wear ear protection *only when needed*.

Use earplugs or earmuffs *only* when:

- sounds around you are uncomfortably loud
- you are around dangerously loud sounds like:
    - lawn mowers
    - loud concerts
    - power tools
    - guns

Is there any research?

Yes. In 2002 Formby, Sherlock, and Gold* studied *sound tolerance.*

- There were two groups of people:
    1. One group wore earplugs for 2 weeks
    2. The other group wore in-the-ear noise generators (maskers) that make a "shhh" sound

- After 2 weeks:
    - The people who wore earplugs could tolerate *less* sound than before
    - The people who wore maskers could tolerate *more* sound than before

- This study showed that:
    - Adding sound makes it easier to tolerate sound
    - Staying in quiet makes it harder to tolerate sound

Bottom line

If everyday sounds bother you:

- Surrounding yourself with comfortable sound will help
- Avoiding sound will make the problem worse

How long does it take?

It can take weeks or months for your ears to adjust.

Talk to your audiologist if you have any questions.

*Formby, C., Sherlock, L.P., & Gold, S.L. (2002). Adaptive calibration of chronic auditory gain: Interim findings. In R. Patuzzi (Ed.), Proceedings of the VIIth International Tinnitus Seminar (pp. 165-69). Crawley: University of Western Australia.

APPENDIX E
Effects of Tinnitus

Tinnitus can have many effects on a person's life. Although there are seemingly hundreds of different effects caused by tinnitus, each can be grouped into one or more of three categories: (1) difficulty concentrating, (2) emotional reactions, and (3) disrupted sleep. Usually, effects of tinnitus include emotional reactions. For example, difficulty concentrating can lead to frustration and anger.

Tinnitus Can Affect Concentration

Imagine you are sitting in a quiet office writing a report. Off in the distance a car alarm goes off. You notice it, but car alarms seem to go off all the time so you don't pay much attention to it. If the alarm continues, however, the sound might distract you from your work. Constant tinnitus is like an "endless car alarm." The sound is not welcome. It cannot be turned off. The challenge is to function in spite of the unwelcome sound.

People are different in their ability to ignore certain sounds. For example, some students like to study with the TV on while others need quiet. Likewise, people are different in the way they ignore tinnitus. For some, it is easy to ignore, while for others it's a distracting sound. When tinnitus distracts you, it can affect any task that needs concentration, such as reading, writing, studying, learning, or problem-solving.

Tinnitus does not make it more difficult to hear. It can, however, *indirectly* affect our hearing if it affects our concentration. It can interfere with focused listening. For that reason, tinnitus can affect our ability to communicate with others.

Tinnitus Can Cause Emotional Reactions

At first, the sound from a car alarm is distracting. If the sound persists, it can become *annoying*. This type of cycle can happen with tinnitus. Emotional reactions can include frustration, worry, and anger. Some people report anxiety or depression because of tinnitus. As mentioned above, effects of tinnitus usually include emotional reactions. For this reason, tinnitus management should focus on managing *reactions* to tinnitus.

Tinnitus Can Disrupt Sleep

People with tinnitus often experience sleep problems. Recall the discussion of contrast reduction on pages 19 and 20. "The sharp contrast between tinnitus and a quiet room attracts attention." When you go to bed at night, you usually are in a quiet room. This situation can make it very difficult to ignore tinnitus. Being aware of tinnitus can make it hard to *fall* asleep. It can also make it hard to *return* to sleep if you wake up in the middle of the night. If tinnitus disrupts sleep each night, you may become sleep deprived. This can make it harder to function normally throughout the day.

If sleep is a problem for you because of tinnitus, please review pages 19 and 20. It is especially important to note how using sound can help you sleep: "Adding sound to the room *reduces the contrast* between the tinnitus and the background. The tinnitus might be just as loud as it was before adding sound to the room. However, *it is easier for the brain to ignore the tinnitus because there is other sound in the room.*" Also, Appendix I offers "tips for getting better sleep."

Why Does Tinnitus Become a Problem?

We discussed *how* tinnitus can become a problem. Now we will discuss *why* it becomes a problem.

1   Many patients report that their tinnitus "came out of nowhere." The tinnitus is a new sound. The new sound can be surprising, and it comes from inside the head - that *really* gets our attention.

2   If the tinnitus is perceived as a *threat*, it will *keep* our attention. Tinnitus can be perceived as a threat if it evokes fears of a serious medical or psychological problem. Patients often report worries that tinnitus means that they "have a tumor" or "are going crazy."

3   We are all different in how we react to sound. The exact same tinnitus sound might bother one person and not another person.

4   Some people say that their tinnitus annoys them because it's always there. The sound is *persistent*, like a dripping water faucet. "Peace and quiet" no longer seems an option.

5   Tinnitus can *trigger negative memories* if the onset of the tinnitus was associated with a traumatic event. The tinnitus may first be noticed following a car accident, a head injury, combat trauma, or a nearby

explosion. Or, it first may be noticed during a time of extreme stress. Thinking about the tinnitus at a later time can trigger these negative memories.

6　Any unwanted sound will become more annoying if it is made louder. A louder sound is harder to ignore. People who report very loud tinnitus seem to be the most bothered by it.

7　The more you pay attention to tinnitus, the more it tends to be a problem. Your lifestyle can affect how much attention is given to tinnitus. Lifestyle factors that may tend to make you pay more attention to tinnitus include: (a) lack of challenging and meaningful activities; (b) spending time in quiet settings; (c) stress; (d) lack of sleep; and (e) unemployment.

8　*Lack of control* is one more reason why tinnitus can become a problem. Even people with mild tinnitus feel that they can't control it or escape it. We want to turn it off, but we don't have that control. We can become frustrated, discouraged, and angry about our lack of control over the sound that's inside our head.

We talked about the car alarm in the distance becoming increasingly bothersome. The alarm becomes a problem when it is *someone else's* car, and you have no control over it. If it is *your own* car you would be able to turn off the alarm and end the problem. This difference in how you react depends on whether or not you feel that you have control.

(Portions of this appendix adapted from Henry, Zaugg, & Schechter, Clinical guide for audiologic tinnitus management II: Treatment. American Journal of Audiology, 14:49-70, 2005)

APPENDIX F
Effects of Hearing Loss

The most common type of hearing loss is "high frequency" loss. This by and large results from loud noise and/or aging. High-frequency hearing is more prone to damage than hearing at lower pitches. A common symptom of high-frequency hearing loss is trouble understanding speech in background noise. If you have hearing loss, hearing aids can help you hear better and may provide relief from stress and tension caused by tinnitus (see Appendix C). If you have trouble hearing, please talk to an audiologist.

Why Does Background Noise Cause Hearing Problems?

With a high-frequency hearing loss, background noise can make it hard to hear clearly. This is because the consonant sounds (for example "t-," "f-," "s-") are high frequency, low energy sounds. They are covered up, or "masked," by other sounds. Vowels are low frequency, high-energy sounds that are not easily masked. You need to hear consonant sounds clearly to tell apart words that sound almost the same, such as "toy" and "soy." It is easy for background sound to "mask out" consonant sounds.

Hearing Loss Creeps Up Slowly

Hearing loss usually creeps up slowly. When this occurs, the first sign is trouble hearing what people are saying in background noise. Often other people will notice the hearing loss before the person who has the hearing loss.

Blaming Hearing Problems on Tinnitus

You might blame recent hearing problems on your tinnitus. As hearing worsens over time, you may get more and more annoyed by the tinnitus. Each time a listening problem occurs, your attention might shift to the tinnitus as the cause. This could result in more attention paid to the tinnitus. This could then lead to an emotional response (for example, frustration or anger). Such thinking can prevail until the hearing loss is detected. But you will have made a *habit of reacting negatively to the tinnitus*. This is how many people develop a problem with their tinnitus.

(Portions of this appendix adapted from Henry, Zaugg, & Schechter, Clinical guide for audiologic tinnitus management II: Treatment. American Journal of Audiology, 14:49-70, 2005)

APPENDIX G
Examples of How People Use Sound to Manage Reactions to Tinnitus

Sound Can be Used in *Many* Ways

There are many examples of *common* ways of using sound to manage tinnitus. There are also *unusual* ways to use sound. Some of these examples are not what you might expect, but they work for some people. *Be open to using sound in unusual or unexpected ways to manage your tinnitus.* (Appendix J shows websites that offer many products for using sound.)

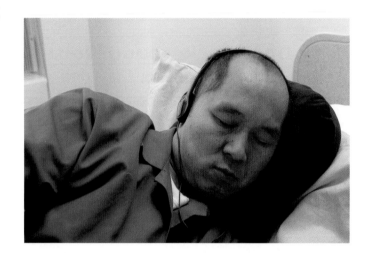

Examples of *Soothing* Sound

Using Environmental Sound as Soothing Sound

	Environmental	Music	Speech
Soothing	✓		
Background			
Interesting			

Carmen notices her tinnitus a lot in her quiet office. The tinnitus annoys her and makes it hard to concentrate. Carmen feels soothed by the sound of ocean waves. When she keeps the sound of ocean waves in her office (using a CD player), she feels better and can concentrate on her work.

Using Music as Soothing Sound

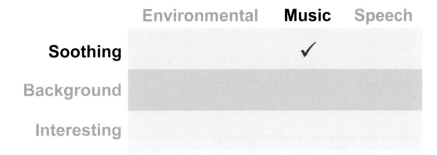

Most mornings Julie woke up feeling irritated that tinnitus was the first sound of the day. She did not like to start her day feeling that way. She started listening to relaxing music every morning when she first woke up. The music gives her a sense of relief and helps her start the day feeling more calm and relaxed.

Using Speech as Soothing Sound

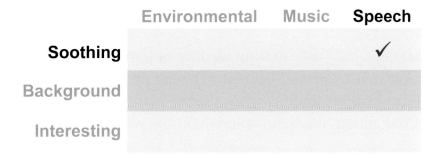

Malcolm listens to audio recordings of relaxation exercises including deep breathing and imagery to get relief from the tension caused by his tinnitus.

What is Imagery?

- *Imagery* is used to help people relax (see p. 38)
- It is done by asking people to close their eyes and picture a peaceful setting
- Imagery is used to relax during stress and as a distraction from tinnitus
- Usually, people feel more relaxed within 5-10 minutes
- The DVD and the CD in the back of this workbook have recordings of an imagery exercise

What is Deep Breathing?

- *Deep breathing* is used to help people relax (see p. 38)

- Deep breathing involves paying careful attention to breathing from the abdomen
- Deep breathing also involves keeping the breath regular and rhythmic
- The DVD and the CD in the back of this workbook have recordings of a deep breathing exercise

Examples of Background Sound

Using Environmental Sound as Background Sound

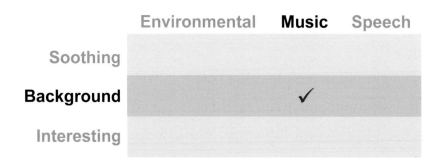

William was having a hard time getting to sleep at night because of his tinnitus. He started running a box fan near his bed. The fan does not give him a sense of relief. He still can hear his tinnitus when the fan is running, but the tinnitus doesn't keep his attention like it did when the room was quiet.

Using Music as Background Sound

Mary's tinnitus made it difficult for her to concentrate on paperwork. She now plays classical music when doing paperwork. The music doesn't make her feel better, and she doesn't pay attention to it. But playing the music helps her to concentrate.

Using Speech as Background Sound

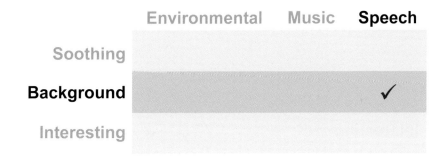

Enrique needed to concentrate in his quiet office but was irritated by his tinnitus. He tried different background sounds on CD, including "crowd noise" (many people talking at once). The crowd noise didn't relax him or make him feel better. But, after a while, he realized that he wasn't thinking about his tinnitus nearly as often as he did when his office was silent.

Examples of Interesting Sound

Using Environmental Sound as Interesting Sound

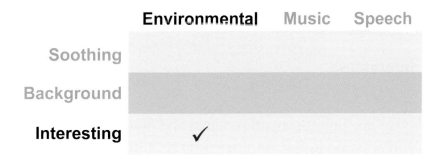

Ben enjoys listening to bird calls. He can identify many local birds by their calls. Sometimes, when his tinnitus is bothering him, he sits on his back porch and listens to bird calls. Other times he goes on-line to learn new bird calls. Actively listening to bird calls gets Ben's mind off of the tinnitus.

Using Music as Interesting Sound

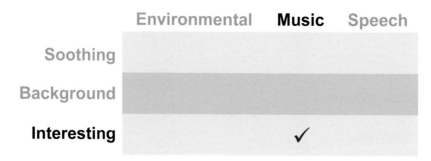

David had trouble relaxing in the evening because his tinnitus was annoying. He started actively listening to the lyrics of songs on his favorite radio station. Paying attention to music lyrics gets his mind off of the tinnitus, which helps him to relax.

Using Speech as Interesting Sound

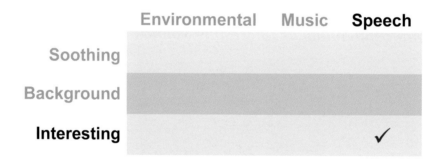

Jane doesn't notice her tinnitus as often when she listens to a book on tape. The book on tape is interesting to her, and listening to it makes it easier to ignore the tinnitus.

APPENDIX H
How to Choose Devices
(To Help with #4 on the Sound Plan
Worksheet)

When filling out #4 on the Sound Plan Worksheet, you can choose from many different devices for getting sound into your ears. We will now give you ideas to help you make your choices. It can help to think of two different *categories* of devices.

1 Wearable Listening Devices
2 Stationary (Tabletop) Devices

Wearable Listening Devices

Wearable listening devices include radios, CD players, cassette tape players, and MP3 players. Some cell phones (like the Apple iPhone) play music. Others have radios built in. Wearable listening devices can be used to manage your tinnitus in almost any setting. If you need hearing aids, then there are options to connect hearing aids with wearable listening devices (described later).

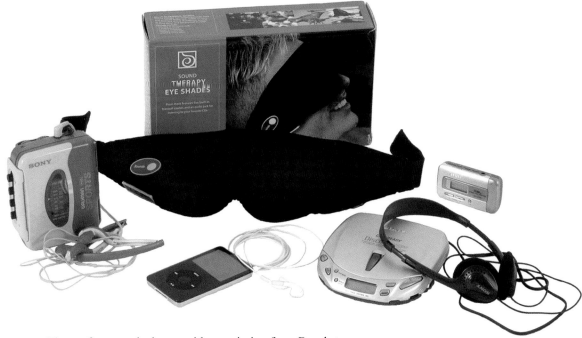

Photo of eye mask shown with permission from Brookstone
Photo of Sony cassette player, CD player and Aiwa radio shown with permission from Sony, Inc.
Photo of iPod shown with permission from Apple, Inc.

MP3 Players

MP3 players (like the Apple iPod) are very flexible listening devices. They can store digital sound files for music, nature sounds, podcasts - whatever you like to listen to. "Earbuds" (in-the-ear earphones) usually are used with MP3 players, although regular earphones also can be used. Some MP3 players double as radios and even cell phones, which makes them even more useful. MP3 players are ideal for listening to special tinnitus-relief sounds that are available on CD.[31] You can use an MP3 player to take sound almost anywhere you need it for your tinnitus.

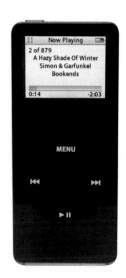

Photo of iPod shown with permission from Apple, Inc.

Bluetooth

Some models of MP3 players offer Bluetooth wireless options. This can make MP3 players more comfortable and convenient to use. Bluetooth is short-range radio technology. It normally is used with cell phones. It allows cell phone users to wear a hands-free earpiece that has a wireless connection with the phone. You can use a wireless earpiece in one or both ears to listen to a Bluetooth-enabled MP3 player worn on a belt or carried in a purse.

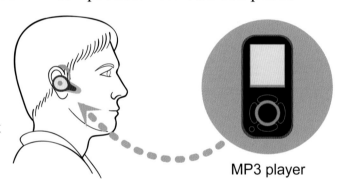

MP3 player

Bluetooth with Hearing Aids

Some behind-the-ear hearing aids have adapters to use with Bluetooth. For tinnitus, this hearing aid and adapter set-up can be used to receive signals directly from Bluetooth-enabled MP3 players.

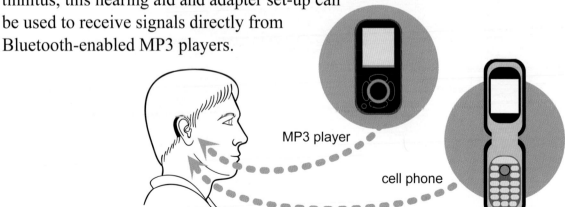

MP3 player

cell phone

Any recorded sound on the MP3 player can be sent directly to your hearing aids with no wires. Signals from Bluetooth-enabled cell phones also can be transmitted to the hearing aids without wires. This results in improved speech understanding while using a cell phone.[32]

Hearing Aids with T-coils

A telephone coil (t-coil) is a tiny coil of wire built into many hearing aids. The t-coil is usually used to pick up inductive (magnetic) signals from telephones. Hearing aids with t-coils also can receive wireless signals from an MP3 player. A neckloop or inductive earhooks can be plugged into the headphone jack of any MP3 player. The signal from the MP3 player is wirelessly transmitted to the t-coil of the hearing aid from the neckloop or earhooks. For some MP3 players, an amplified neckloop may be needed. Signals from cell phones with standard headphone jacks also can be transmitted to t-coils using a neckloop or inductive earhooks. This allows wireless delivery of sound from any audio device with a standard headphone jack direct to any hearing aid t-coil.

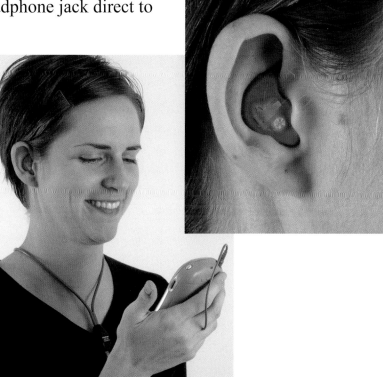

Satellite Radio

Satellite Radio offers many listening choices. About 160 channels are available. A special receiver is needed (average price around $100) along with monthly service (about $10/month). Each receiver has different features. Some receivers can store hours of programs for later listening. The main advantage of Satellite Radio is the large number of listening choices.

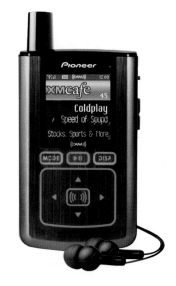

Photo of satellite radio courtesy of Pioneeer Electronics (USA) Inc.

Stationary Listening Devices

Stationary listening devices include:

- Tabletop sound generators
- CD players
- Radios
- MP3 "docking stations"
- Tabletop fountains

These devices are useful in quiet rooms such as offices and bedrooms. Stationary listening devices help "enrich" your sound environment. They can be used even if you use hearing aids or ear-level noise generators. (Appendix J shows websites that offer a variety of stationary listening devices.)

Benefits of Stationary Listening Devices

Any sound that you can listen to with *wearable* listening devices also works with *stationary* listening devices. CDs can be played on many kinds of systems. MP3 players can be used in docking stations for tabletop use. Cassette tapes, although no longer popular, are still options - especially for music and talk formats. Radios offer many program choices. Satellite Radio is available in tabletop models. Tabletop water fountains and electric fans provide steady background sound. Any of these devices can be useful in a quiet setting where you spend time. They are helpful in the office, bedroom, and reading areas.

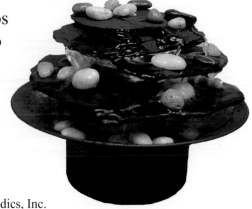

Photo of tabletop fountain shown with permission from HoMedics, Inc.

If you have trouble sleeping because of tinnitus, a tabletop sound device next to the bed may help. "Sound pillows" offer another listening choice.

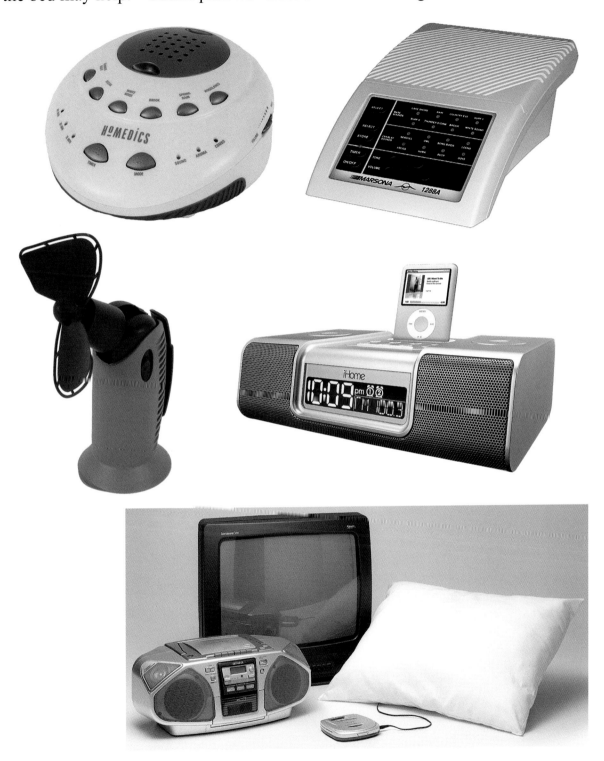

Photo of Marsona sound machine courtesy of Marpac Corporation
Photo of HoMedics sound machine shown with permission from HoMedics, Inc.
Photo of iHome radio and docking station courtesy of KIDdesigns, Inc.
Photo of Sound Pillow courtesy of Phoenix Productions & Promotional Products

Sight and Sound

Using both sight and sound can be very useful to get your thoughts off of your tinnitus. Options include movies (theatre, DVD, VHS), TV shows, plays, concerts, and comedy club. The content should always be *meaningful* and *interesting* to you - to keep your attention.

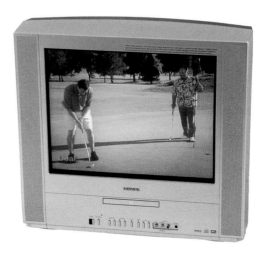

Also, there are special DVDs that show peaceful scenes with relaxing music in the background.

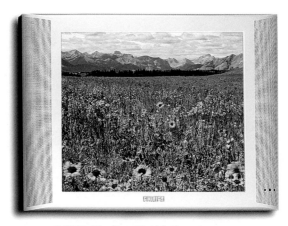

©2008 Healing HealthCare Systems

Photo of Toshiba TV shown with permission from Brodeur Partners

APPENDIX I
Tips for Getting Better Sleep

Sleep is essential to good health. Sleep helps your body to repair itself, both physically and emotionally. Your tinnitus may seem worse when you are tired. When you get enough sleep, you are ready to handle problems and you won't get frustrated as easily. A good night's sleep will give you energy to practice skills from this workbook.[20]

What happens if you don't get enough sleep?

- Your tinnitus may seem louder
- Problems seem more difficult to handle
- Your body feels weak
- You don't feel good or enjoy activities
- You have difficulty concentrating

Tips for sleeping well:

Timing:

- Set the alarm and get up at the same time everyday (regardless of how much you slept)
- Do not nap during the day, or limit your naps to no more than 30 minutes each day (unless you have been advised differently by your doctor)
- Go to bed at the same time each day

Sleep Behavior:

- Go to bed only when sleepy
- Use the bed and bedroom only for sleep (do not read, eat, or watch TV in bed)
- If unable to sleep - get out of bed
- Don't lie in bed awake for more than 20 minutes - get up
- Engage in a quiet activity - return to bed when sleepy
- Repeat the above strategy for as many times as is necessary

- Teach your body to associate the bed with sleep, not frustration

- Only spend the amount of time in bed that you want to spend sleeping even if you did not sleep as well or as much as you would have liked. For example, if you want seven hours of sleep then only spend seven hours in bed.

- Don't sleep in or nap more than usual because you didn't sleep well the night before

Body Temperature:

- Increasing your body temperature during the day can help you sleep better at night

- Don't exercise or bathe too close to bedtime

- You can raise body temperature by exercising a few hours before bed

- You can raise body temperature by taking a warm bath for about 30 minutes about two hours before bedtime

The Bedroom:

- Keep the same temperature in the bedroom throughout the night; make sure that the temperature is not too warm.

- Overheating can disrupt deep sleep

- Brightly lit wall clocks can disrupt sleep

- Keep the room dark. (Note: A night light may be needed to safely get up in the night to go to the restroom without falling.)

- Develop a "sound plan" to learn how to use sound to manage your tinnitus at night (see p. 27).
    - Also use constant low-level sound to keep other sounds from waking you up. (See Appendix J for websites that offer tabletop sound machines.)

Effort and Sleep:

- Making an "effort" to fall asleep will not help you sleep

- Sleep should not be effortful

- Avoid mentally stimulating activity just before going to bed. For example, don't watch an action movie or have really interesting conversation just before bedtime.

- Relaxation techniques such as deep breathing and visual imagery can help you get to sleep or back to sleep when you awaken in the night
- Mentally quiet tasks such as listening to music and calming thoughts can help you relax and sleep

Diet:
- Caffeine (a stimulant) should be discontinued at least 4-6 hours before bedtime*
- Nicotine (a stimulant) should be avoided near bedtime and when you awaken in the night*
- Alcohol (a depressant) causes awakenings later in the night even though it might have helped you fall asleep*
- A light snack may be sleep-inducing but a heavy meal too close to bedtime might interfere with sleep

Check with your doctor before using any of these substances

More information about sleep is available from Patlak, M. (November, 2005). U.S. Department of Health and Human Services; National Institutes of Health; National Heart, Lung, and Blood Institute. *Your Guide to Healthy Sleep*. NIH Publication No. 06-5271. (available as a free download from http://www.nhlbi.nih.gov/health/public/sleep/healthy_sleep.htm)

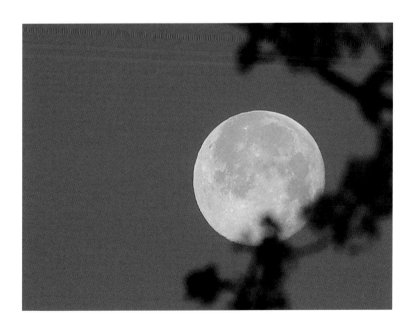

APPENDIX J
Resources

"Knowledge is power." Learning about tinnitus can help you manage it and control your reactions to it. There are many good books and websites about tinnitus. Be aware that some websites have wrong or misleading information. Contact your audiologist if you have any questions.

Websites (Websites accessed January 16, 2010; this list does not comprise an endorsement of any of these products or companies)

Websites to Locate Therapeutic Sounds and Sound-Producing Devices

Sites for CDs and Downloads

www.sleepmachines.com

www.serenitysupply.com

www.binaural.com/bines.html

www.naturesound.com

www.purewhitenoise.com

www.empoweredwithin.com

www.audiobooks.com

www.npr.org/podcast

www.audiobionics.com

Other Sound Devices

www.bizrate.com

www.water-fountain.biz

www.simplyfountains.com

www.overstock.com

www.sirius.com

www.soundpillow.com

www.healinghealth.com

Tabletop Sound-Generating Devices

www.brookstone.com

www.catalogclearance.com

www.marpac.com

www.soundtherapyworld.com

www.homedics.com

www.naturestapestry.com

www.soundmachinesdirect.com

www.adcohearing.com

www.halhen.com

Ear-level Tinnitus Instruments

www.generalhearing.com

www.amplisound.com

www.widexusa.com

www.gnresound.com

www.beltone.com

Websites for Information About Tinnitus

www.ncrar.research.va.gov

www.ata.org

www.tinnitus.org.uk

www.ohsu.edu/ohrc

www.nidcd.nih.gov/health/hearing/noiseinear.asp

Websites to Locate Products for Hearing Protection

www.earinc.com

www.etymotic.com

www.earplugstore.com

www.howardleight.com

Website for Information about Getting Better Sleep

http://www.nhlbi.nih.gov/health/public/sleep/healthy_sleep.htm

Tinnitus Video

We made a 13-minute video with basic information about tinnitus. You can watch it on your computer via the NCRAR website (http://www.ncrar.research. va.gov/ForVets/Resources.asp). If it does not work on your computer, contact the NCRAR and request a copy.

Public Library

You can access the internet for free at a public library. If you don't know how to use the internet, a librarian will show you how. You can use the internet to access the websites listed above. You can also borrow CDs and DVDs from public libraries.

Any advice about tinnitus and hearing disorders given by this workbook is general information. It is not a substitute for proper medical care. No responsibility can be accepted for the outcome on any health problem on which we may have commented in this way.

References

1. Schechter MA, Henry JA. Assessment and treatment of tinnitus patients using a "masking approach." *Journal of the American Academy of Audiology 2002*;13:545-558.

2. Henry JA, Trune DR, Robb MJA, Jastreboff PJ. *Tinnitus Retraining Therapy: Clinical Guidelines*. San Diego: Plural Publishing, Inc.; 2007.

3. Davis PB. Music and the acoustic desensitization protocol for tinnitus. In: Tyler RS, editor. *Tinnitus Treatment: Clinical Protocols*. New York: Thieme Medical Publishers, Inc.; 2006. p. 146-160.

4. Henry JA, Zaugg TL, Schechter MA. Clinical guide for audiologic tinnitus management II: Treatment. *American Journal of Audiology 2005*;14:49-70.

5. Henry JL, Wilson PH. *The Psychological Management of Chronic Tinnitus*. Needham Heights: Allyn & Bacon; 2001.

6. Henry JL, Wilson PH. *Tinnitus: A Self-Management Guide for the Ringing in Your Ears*. Boston: Allyn & Bacon; 2002.

7. Henry JA, Zaugg TL, Myers PJ, Schechter MA. Progressive Audiologic Tinnitus Management. *The Asha Leader 2008*;13(8):14-17.

8. Henry JA, Zaugg TL, Myers PJ, Schechter MA. The role of audiologic evaluation in Progressive Audiologic Tinnitus Management. *Trends in Amplification 2008*;12(3):169-184.

9. Henry JA, Zaugg TL, Myers PJ, Schechter MA. Using therapeutic sound with Progressive Audiologic Tinnitus Management. *Trends in Amplification 2008*;12(3):185-206.

10. Henry JA, Dennis K, Schechter MA. General review of tinnitus: Prevalence, mechanisms, effects, and management. *Journal of Speech, Language, and Hearing Research 2005*;48(5):1204-1234.

11. Beck JS. *Cognitive Therapy: Basics and Beyond*. New York: Guilford; 1995.

12. DiSorga RM. Adverse drug reactions and audiology practice. *Audiology Today 2001*;13(Special Issue: Drug Reactions):2-7.

13. Hazell J. Management of tinnitus. In: Ludman H, Wright T, editors. *Diseases of the Ear*. London: Arnold; 1998. p. 202-215.

14. Perry BP, Gantz BJ. Medical and surgical evaluation and management of tinnitus. In: Tyler RS, editor. *Tinnitus Handbook*. San Diego: Singular Publishing Group; 2000. p. 221-241.

15. Dauman R. Electrical stimulation for tinnitus suppression. In: Tyler R, editor. *Tinnitus Handbook*. San Diego: Singular Publishing Group; 2000. p. 377-398.

16. Folmer RL, Carroll JR, Rahim A, Shi Y, Hal Martin W. Effects of repetitive transcranial magnetic stimulation (rTMS) on chronic tinnitus. *Acta Oto-Laryngologica 2006*;126(Supplement 556):96-101.

17. Langguth B, Hajak G, Kleinjung T, Pridmore S, Sand P, Eichhammer P. Repetitive transcranial magnetic stimulation and chronic tinnitus. *Acta Oto-Laryngologica 2006*;126(Supplement 556):102-4.

18. Londero A, Langguth B, De Ridder D, Bonfils P, Lefaucheur JP. Repetitive transcranial magnetic stimulation (rTMS): a new therapeutic approach in subjective tinnitus? *Neurophysiol Clin 2006*;36(3):145-55.

19. Dobie RA. Clinical trials and drug therapy for tinnitus. In: Snow JB, editor. *Tinnitus: Theory and Management*. Lewiston, NY: BC Decker Inc.; 2004. p. 266-277.

20. Kerns RD, Turk DC, Holzman AD, Rudy TE. Comparison of cognitive-behavioral and behavioral approaches to the outpatient treatment of chronic pain. *Clinical Journal of Pain 1986*;1:195-203.

21. Henry JA, Schechter MA, Nagler SM, Fausti SA. Comparison of Tinnitus Masking and Tinnitus Retraining Therapy. *Journal of the American Academy of Audiology 2002*;13:559-581.

22. Vernon JA, Meikle MB. Tinnitus masking. In: Tyler RS, editor. *Tinnitus Handbook*. San Diego: Singular Publishing Group; 2000. p. 313-356.

23. Henry JA, Trune DR, Robb MJA, Jastreboff PJ. *Tinnitus Retraining Therapy: Patient Counseling Guide*. San Diego: Plural Publishing, Inc.; 2007.

24. Jastreboff PJ. The neurophysiological model of tinnitus. In: Snow JB, editor. *Tinnitus: Theory and Management*. Lewiston, NY: BC Decker Inc.; 2004. p. 96-107.

25. Jastreboff PJ. Tinnitus habituation therapy (THT) and tinnitus retraining therapy (TRT). In: Tyler RS, editor. *Tinnitus Handbook*. San Diego: Singular Publishing Group; 2000. p. 357-376.

26. Jastreboff PJ, Hazell JWP. *Tinnitus Retraining Therapy: Implementing the Neurophysiological Model*. New York: Cambridge University Press; 2004.

27. Davis PB, Wilde RA, Steed LG. Trials of Tinnitus Desensitisation Music: neurophysiology-influenced rehabilitation. In: Patuzzi R, editor. *Proceedings of the Seventh International Tinnitus Seminar*. Crawley: The University of Western Australia; 2002. p. 74-77.

28. Henry JA, Zaugg TL, Myers PJ, Kendall CJ, Turbin MB. Principles and application of counseling used in Progressive Audiologic Tinnitus Management. *Noise and Health 2009*;11(42):33-48.

29. Drew S, Davies E. Effectiveness of Ginkgo biloba in treating tinnitus: double blind, placebo controlled trial. *Bmj 2001*;322(7278):73.

30. Dobie RA. A review of randomized clinical trials in tinnitus. *The Laryngoscope 1999*;109:1202-1211.

31. Henry JA, Rheinsburg B, Zaugg T. Comparison of custom sounds for achieving tinnitus relief. *Journal of the American Academy of Audiology 2004*;15:585-598.

32. Tchorz J. Utilizing Bluetooth for better speech understanding over the cell phone. *The Hearing Review 2005*;12(1):50-51.

Sound Plan Worksheet

1. Write down one bothersome tinnitus situation _____

2. **Check one or more** of the three ways to use sound to manage the situation	3. **Write down the sounds** that you will try	4. **Write down the devices** you will use	5. Use your sound plan **over the next week. How helpful** was each sound after using it for 1 week?	6. **Comments** When you find something that works well (or not so well) please comment. You do not need to wait 1 week to write your comments.
☐ **Soothing sound** (TINNITUS — Soft breezes, Soothing voice, Babbling brook, Relaxing music, Running water, Ocean waves)	_____	_____	Not at all / A little / Moderately / Very much / Extremely (☐ ☐ ☐ ☐ ☐)	_____
☐ **Background sound** (TINNITUS — Other Sound Other Sound, Other Sound Other Sound, Other Sound Other Sound, Other Sound Other Sound and Other)	_____	_____	Not at all / A little / Moderately / Very much / Extremely (☐ ☐ ☐ ☐ ☐)	_____
☐ **Interesting sound** (TINNITUS — Talk Radio!, Audio Books!)	_____	_____	Not at all / A little / Moderately / Very much / Extremely (☐ ☐ ☐ ☐ ☐)	_____

Changing Thoughts and Feelings Worksheet

1. From the Tinnitus Problem Checklist, write down one bothersome tinnitus situation _____

2. **Check one or more** of the three skills to manage the situation	3. **Write down the details** for each skill you will use	4. **Use your plan** over the next week. **How helpful** was each exercise?	5. **Comments** When you find something that works well (or not so well) please comment. You do not need to wait 1 week to write your comments.

☐ **Relaxation exercises**

breathe		
Relax		
imagine		

☐ Deep breathing _____ ☐ Not at all ☐ A little ☐ Moderately ☐ Very much ☐ Extremely

☐ Imagery _____ ☐ Not at all ☐ A little ☐ Moderately ☐ Very much ☐ Extremely

☐ Other _____ ☐ Not at all ☐ A little ☐ Moderately ☐ Very much ☐ Extremely

☐ **Plan pleasant activities**

golf, write, walk Activity 1 _____
Pleasant activities Activity 2 _____
dance, paint Activity 3 _____

Activity 1 ☐ Not at all ☐ A little ☐ Moderately ☐ Very much ☐ Extremely
Activity 2 ☐ Not at all ☐ A little ☐ Moderately ☐ Very much ☐ Extremely
Activity 3 ☐ Not at all ☐ A little ☐ Moderately ☐ Very much ☐ Extremely

_____
_____
_____

☐ **Changing thoughts**

Think → *Feel*

Old thought _____
_____

New thought _____
_____

☐ Not at all ☐ A little ☐ Moderately ☐ Very much ☐ Extremely

_____
_____
_____

Sound Plan Worksheet

1. Write down one bothersome tinnitus situation _____

2. Check one or more of the three ways to use sound to manage the situation

3. Write down the sounds that you will try

4. Write down the devices you will use

5. Use your sound plan **over the next week. How helpful** was each sound after using it for 1 week?

6. Comments
When you find something that works well (or not so well) please comment. You do not need to wait 1 week to write your comments.

☐ **Soothing sound**

(Soft breeze
Soothing voice
Babbling brook
TINNITUS
Relaxing music
Running water
Ocean waves)

Not at all A little Moderately Very much Extremely
☐ ☐ ☐ ☐ ☐
☐ ☐ ☐ ☐ ☐
☐ ☐ ☐ ☐ ☐

☐ **Background sound**

(Other Sound Other Sou...
...her Sound Other Sou...
TINNITUS
...Other Sound Other So...
t Other Sound Oth...
...ound and Oth...)

Not at all A little Moderately Very much Extremely
☐ ☐ ☐ ☐ ☐
☐ ☐ ☐ ☐ ☐
☐ ☐ ☐ ☐ ☐

☐ **Interesting sound**

(Talk
Radio!
TINNITUS
Audio
Books!)

Not at all A little Moderately Very much Extremely
☐ ☐ ☐ ☐ ☐
☐ ☐ ☐ ☐ ☐
☐ ☐ ☐ ☐ ☐

Changing Thoughts and Feelings Worksheet

1. From the Tinnitus Problem Checklist, write down one bothersome tinnitus situation _____

2. Check one or more of the three skills to manage the situation

3. Write down the details for each skill you will use

4. Use your plan over the next week. **How helpful** was each exercise?

5. Comments When you find something that works well (or not so well) please comment. You do not need to wait 1 week to write your comments.

☐ **Relaxation exercises**

	breathe	
Relax		
imagine		

☐ Deep breathing _____

☐ Imagery _____

☐ Other _____

Not at all | A little | Moderately | Very much | Extremely
☐ ☐ ☐ ☐ ☐
☐ ☐ ☐ ☐ ☐
☐ ☐ ☐ ☐ ☐

_____
_____
_____

☐ **Plan pleasant activities**

golf, write, walk

Pleasant activities

dance, paint

Activity 1 _____
Activity 2 _____
Activity 3 _____

Not at all | A little | Moderately | Very much | Extremely
☐ ☐ ☐ ☐ ☐
☐ ☐ ☐ ☐ ☐
☐ ☐ ☐ ☐ ☐

_____
_____
_____

☐ **Changing thoughts**

Old thought _____

New thought _____

Not at all | A little | Moderately | Very much | Extremely
☐ ☐ ☐ ☐ ☐

_____
_____
_____

Think → Feel

Sound Plan Worksheet

1. Write down one bothersome tinnitus situation _____

2. Check one or more of the three ways to use sound to manage the situation

3. Write down the sounds that you will try

4. Write down the devices you will use

5. Use your sound plan over the next week. How helpful was each sound after using it for 1 week?

Not at all · A little · Moderately · Very much · Extremely

6. Comments When you find something that works well (or not so well) please comment. You do not need to wait 1 week to write your comments.

☐ **Soothing sound**

(TINNITUS — Soft breezes, Soothing voice, Babbling brook, Relaxing music, Running water, Ocean waves)

☐ **Background sound**

(TINNITUS — Sound Other, Other Sound Other Sound, Other Sound Other Sound, Other Sound Other Sound, Other Sound Other Sound, Sound Other)

☐ **Interesting sound**

(TINNITUS — Talk Radio!, Audio Books!)

Changing Thoughts and Feelings Worksheet

1. From the Tinnitus Problem Checklist, write down one bothersome tinnitus situation _____

2. **Check one or more** of the three skills to manage the situation

☐ **Relaxation exercises**

	breathe
Relax	
imagine	

☐ Deep breathing

☐ Imagery

☐ Other _____

☐ **Plan pleasant activities**

golf, write, walk

Pleasant activities

dance, paint

Activity 1

Activity 2

Activity 3

☐ **Changing thoughts**

Old thought

New thought

Think ← Feel

3. **Write down the details** for each skill you will use

_____

_____

_____

_____

_____

_____

_____

_____

_____

4. **Use your plan** over the next week. **How helpful** was each exercise?

Not at all / A little / Moderately / Very much / Extremely

☐ ☐ ☐ ☐ ☐
☐ ☐ ☐ ☐ ☐
☐ ☐ ☐ ☐ ☐

Not at all / A little / Moderately / Very much / Extremely

☐ ☐ ☐ ☐ ☐
☐ ☐ ☐ ☐ ☐
☐ ☐ ☐ ☐ ☐

Not at all / A little / Moderately / Very much / Extremely

☐ ☐ ☐ ☐ ☐

5. **Comments** When you find something that works well (or not so well) please comment. You do not need to wait 1 week to write your comments.

_____

_____

_____

_____

_____

Sound Plan Worksheet

1. Write down one bothersome tinnitus situation

2. **Check one or more** of the three ways to use sound to manage the situation

3. **Write down the sounds** that you will try

4. **Write down the devices** you will use

5. Use your sound plan **over the next week. How helpful** was each sound after using it for 1 week?

6. **Comments**
When you find something that works well (or not so well) please comment. You do not need to wait 1 week to write your comments.

☐ **Soothing sound**

TINNITUS
Soft breezes
Soothing voice
Babbling brook
Relaxing music
Running water
Ocean waves

Not at all | A little | Moderately | Very much | Extremely

☐ **Background sound**

TINNITUS
Other Sound Other So
ther Sound Other Soun
ther Sound Other Sound
Other Sound Other Sou
r Other Sound Oth
sound Other

Not at all | A little | Moderately | Very much | Extremely

☐ **Interesting sound**

TINNITUS
Talk
Radio!
Audio
Books!

Not at all | A little | Moderately | Very much | Extremely

Changing Thoughts and Feelings Worksheet

1. From the Tinnitus Problem Checklist, write down one bothersome tinnitus situation _____

2. **Check one or more** of the three skills to manage the situation

☐ **Relaxation exercises**

breathe
Relax
imagine

☐ Deep breathing

☐ Imagery

☐ Other _____

☐ **Plan pleasant activities**

golf, write, walk
Pleasant activities
dance, paint

Activity 1 _____

Activity 2 _____

Activity 3 _____

☐ **Changing thoughts**

Think → Feel

Old thought _____

New thought _____

3. **Write down the details** for each skill you will use

4. **Use your plan** over the next week. When you find something that works well (or not so well) please comment. You do not need to wait 1 week to write your comments.

How helpful was each exercise?

☐ Not at all
☐ A little
☐ Moderately
☐ Very much
☐ Extremely

☐☐☐ Not at all
☐☐☐ A little
☐☐☐ Moderately
☐☐☐ Very much
☐☐☐ Extremely

☐ Not at all
☐ A little
☐ Moderately
☐ Very much
☐ Extremely

5. **Comments**
_____
_____
_____

Sound Plan Worksheet

1. Write down one bothersome tinnitus situation _____

2. Check one or more of the three ways to use sound to manage the situation

3. Write down the sounds that you will try

4. Write down the devices you will use

5. Use your sound plan **over the next week. How helpful** was each sound after using it for 1 week?

6. **Comments** When you find something that works well (or not so well) please comment. You do not need to wait 1 week to write your comments.

☐ **Soothing sound**

(TINNITUS / Soft breezes / Soothing voice / Bubbling brook / Relaxing music / Running water / Ocean waves)

Not at all | A little | Moderately | Very much | Extremely

☐ **Background sound**

(TINNITUS / Sound Other / ...Sound Other Sou... / ...er Sound Other Soun... / ...ther Sound Other Soun... / Other Sound Other Sou... / r Other Sound Oth... / ...und and Oth...)

Not at all | A little | Moderately | Very much | Extremely

☐ **Interesting sound**

(TINNITUS / Talk Radio! / Audio Books!)

Not at all | A little | Moderately | Very much | Extremely

Changing Thoughts and Feelings Worksheet

1. From the Tinnitus Problem Checklist, write down one bothersome tinnitus situation _____

2. **Check one or more** of the three skills to manage the situation

☐ **Relaxation exercises**

breathe
Relax
imagine

☐ Deep breathing

☐ Imagery

☐ Other

☐ **Plan pleasant activities**

golf, write, walk
Pleasant activities
dance, paint

Activity 1 _____

Activity 2 _____

Activity 3 _____

☐ **Changing thoughts**

[Think ← Feel]

Old thought _____

New thought _____

3. **Write down the details** for each skill you will use

4. **Use your plan** over the next week. **How helpful** was each exercise?

☐ Not at all ☐ A little ☐ Moderately ☐ Very much ☐ Extremely

☐ Not at all ☐ A little ☐ Moderately ☐ Very much ☐ Extremely

☐ Not at all ☐ A little ☐ Moderately ☐ Very much ☐ Extremely

☐ Not at all ☐ A little ☐ Moderately ☐ Very much ☐ Extremely

☐ Not at all ☐ A little ☐ Moderately ☐ Very much ☐ Extremely

5. **Comments**
When you find something that works well (or not so well) please comment. You do not need to wait 1 week to write your comments.

_____
_____
_____

_____
_____
_____

Descriptions of DVD and Audio CD

A DVD and a CD are attached to the back cover of this workbook. The DVD contains four videos. The first two videos are about using sound to manage reactions to tinnitus. The third and fourth videos are about two relaxation techniques. The third video shows "deep breathing." The fourth video shows "imagery." With the audio CD, a speaker explains how sound can be used to manage reactions to tinnitus. The CD also includes sound tracks that demonstrate many uses of sound for tinnitus.

Managing Your Tinnitus DVD

Managing Your Tinnitus, Session 1

Length: 35:38

This is the first of two videos about using sound to manage reactions to tinnitus. In this video, Drs. Henry and Zaugg explain how to make a customized "sound plan." A sound plan is used to help you when your tinnitus is bothersome.

Managing Your Tinnitus, Session 2

Length: 26:30

This is the second of two videos about using sound to manage reactions to tinnitus. Drs. Henry and Zaugg begin by reviewing the first video. They then explain how to choose listening devices. This is followed by ideas for improving your sound plan. Next, different ways of using sound are reviewed. Finally, they talk about other things you can do to manage your reactions to tinnitus.

Managing Your Tinnitus, Imagery Exercise

Length: 10:19

"Imagery" is another way to relieve stress and tension. This video shows an imagery exercise. This exercise can help you manage your reactions to tinnitus.

Managing Your Tinnitus, Deep Breathing Exercise

Length: 12:48

There is no safe and consistent way to quiet tinnitus. There are, however, many ways to feel better by using techniques that relieve stress and tension. One of these techniques is "deep breathing." This video shows a deep-breathing exercise.

Managing Your Tinnitus Sound Demonstration CD
Total CD length: 01:16:18

TRACK 1	Sound Demo Introduction	1:14
TRACK 2	Types of Sound	6:48
TRACK 3	Environmental Sound, Music, Speech	6:33
TRACK 4	Examples of Soothing Sound	5:05
TRACK 5	Examples of Interesting Sound	2:48
TRACK 6	Examples of Background Sound	3:03
TRACK 7	Sound Demo Close	1:12
TRACK 8	Introduction to Sample Sounds	0:37
TRACK 9	Soothing Sound: Water	1:10
TRACK 10	Soothing Sound: Audio Bionics DTM E-Nature	1:10
TRACK 11	Soothing Sound: Audio Bionics DTM E-Air	1:11
TRACK 12	Soothing Sound: Audio Bionics DTM E-Water	1:12
TRACK 13	Soothing Sound: Music	2:40
TRACK 14	Soothing Sound: Imagery Demonstration	2:25
TRACK 15	Interesting Sound: Urban Legend (from "What Sticks")	1:33
TRACK 16	Interesting Sound: JFK/Apollo 11	1:35
TRACK 17	Interesting Sound: Birds	1:34
TRACK 18	Interesting Sound: Animals	1:50
TRACK 19	Interesting Sound: Music	2:28
TRACK 20	Background Sound: Restaurant	2:22
TRACK 21	Background Sound: City Traffic	2:17
TRACK 22	Background Sound: Elevator Music	2:29
TRACK 23	Background Sound: Fish Tank	2:24
TRACK 24	Introduction to Deep Breathing and Imagery	0:24
TRACK 25	Deep Breathing Exercise	11:19
TRACK 26	Imagery Exercise	8:55